Mutual Support and
Mental Health

Community, Culture and Change
(formerly Therapeutic Communities)
Series editors: Rex Haigh and Jan Lees

Community, Culture and Change encompasses a wide range of ideas and theoretical models related to communities and cultures as a whole, embracing key Therapeutic Community concepts such as collective responsibility, citizenship and empowerment, as well as multidisciplinary ways of working and the social origins of distress. The ways in which our social and therapeutic worlds are changing are illustrated by the innovative and creative work described in these books.

Mutual Support and Mental Health

A Route to Recovery

Maddy Loat

Jessica Kingsley *Publishers*
London and Philadelphia

First published in 2011
by Jessica Kingsley Publishers
116 Pentonville Road
London N1 9JB, UK
and
400 Market Street, Suite 400
Philadelphia, PA 19106, USA

www.jkp.com

Library of Congress Cataloging in Publication Data
A CIP catalogue record for this book is available from the Library of Congress

British Library Cataloguing in Publication Data
A CIP catalogue record for this book is available from the British Library

ISBN 978 1 84310 530 5

Printed and bound in Great Britain

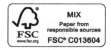

The necessity to unite with other living beings, to be related to them, is an imperative need on the fulfilment of which man's sanity depends.

Erich Fromm, The Sane Society (1956)

Acknowledgements

This book is dedicated to my mother, Thelma, who has always been such an inspiration to me…and who, from ever since I can remember, has provided support and guidance whilst encouraging exploration of new territory and teaching me that this is different to the map.

To my husband Gareth, for his constant support and encouragement, and for his patience and good humour during the writing of this book. Also, for his invaluable editorial work once the book was written.

Wayne, Catherine, Ruben and Anne…for their friendship and support over the years.

I am grateful to Rex Haigh, Jan Lees and everyone involved at Jessica Kingsley Publishers. I deeply appreciate the support of Nancy Pistrang at University College London, who shared her extensive knowledge of mutual support with me during supervision of my research and beyond; and Craig Fees at the Planned Environment Therapy Trust, who generously became a much-needed guide to the therapeutic community world and provided a wealth of information. Also, I should like to thank Kevin Healy, Clinical Director of the Cassel Hospital, for making it possible for me to conduct my research there, and to all those who participated in the study – their stories form the essence of this book.

Last but certainly not least – this book would not have been possible without all the people I have met and learnt from during my time working within mental health, both service users and work colleagues. There are many brave and selfless people that I have had the privilege of getting to know during this time, and I would like to thank them for sharing their stories and their experiences with me.

Contents

INTRODUCTION   9

PART I Processes and Functions of Mutual Support   **15**

1. What Is Mutual Support?   17

2. Mutual Support from a Developmental Perspective   24

3. Mental Health Difficulties and Social Functioning   33

PART II Mutual Support and Mental Health Provision   **43**

4. Formal and Informal Help   45

5. Group Therapy   55

6. Therapeutic Communities   65

PART III Applications of Mutual Support   **79**

7. Does Mutual Support Work? Exploring the Evidence Base   81

8. Putting Theory into Practice: How to Make a Difference   91

9. The Future of Mutual Support   103

   FURTHER INFORMATION   109

   REFERENCES   131

   SUBJECT INDEX   138

   AUTHOR INDEX   142

List of Tables

3.1 Erikson's psychosocial stages of personality development
(Erikson 1968)   35

6.1 Core values for therapeutic communities   75

6.2 Core standards for therapeutic communities   76

7.1 Research findings from exploration of mutual support processes in a
therapeutic community (Loat 2006)   89

List of Figures

5.1 A classification of group methods (Pines and Schlapobersky 2000)   58

Introduction

This book was born out of my experiences working within the field of mental health. During this time I have worked in various capacities and within a diverse range of settings, including statutory and non-statutory services. Although these experiences have been significantly different, there have been a number of common threads running through which have only become visible to me through the passage of time. The pages that follow are my attempt at weaving these threads together.

My first attempt at exploring mutual support and mental health was in 2004 when I researched processes of mutual support and the different ways it influenced individuals who were working through serious and enduring mental health difficulties. These individuals were residents of the Cassel Hospital, one of the oldest and most respected therapeutic communities in the UK. The stories they told me provided evidence that recovery, even from the most traumatic experiences, is possible, but that this tends to be a shared rather than a solitary endeavour.

All mental health services, despite the different approaches they may take, share a common aim in trying to understand and alleviate the difficulties and suffering of those experiencing mental health problems. However, these difficulties are pervasive and cannot be confined within the boundaries of these services, or indeed within the individuals who experience them. The longer I have worked in mental health, the more strongly I hold the view that attempting to understand and treat mental health within these limits is rather like trying to put together a jigsaw puzzle with missing pieces. The book's aim is to help identify and locate these missing pieces, as only then can we start to see the bigger picture and understand more about mental health and what it comprises. In order to do this, I propose that we need to consider how mental health difficulties can be understood and addressed within the context of the social system: in our day-to-day interactions with one another and within the communities that we inhabit.

In my work with adults who are experiencing acute mental health problems I frequently hear stories relating to experiences involving isolation, disempowerment and shame. This is not surprising when we consider the stigma associated with mental health, and although this is slowly reducing we still have a long way to go. My experiences have led me to believe that if we are to understand and treat mental health problems to the best of our abilities, it is necessary to widen our focus beyond the individual to the realm of the interpersonal.

Essentially, humans are social beings – wherever we reside, whether it be alone or surrounded by others, we cannot escape the fundamental truth that we are connected to and depend upon each other in order to survive. Mental health problems frequently correlate with difficulties in social relationships and interpersonal functioning; yet despite this, the majority of mental health services tend to favour an individual-centric approach. This involves viewing and treating mental health difficulties from the perspective that they are located within the individual alone, while the wider social context tends to be overlooked or downplayed.

Early on in my career I was fortunate enough to stumble across the domain of therapeutic communities, and even more fortunate to have the opportunity to work within them for a period of time. This was a truly formative experience that has shaped the way I think about mental health and has had a major influence on the way I approach my clinical work. I discuss therapeutic communities in depth in Chapter 6 but I think it would be useful to say a few words about them here as the approach they take is very much in line with, and fundamental to, the ideas that this book is concerned with.

Therapeutic communities are organisations where a group, or 'community' of people work together therapeutically. The therapeutic community approach involves attempting to understand the individual and the difficulties they are experiencing within the context of the group or community of which they are part. Underlying this is a belief that who we are is dependent upon and constituted by our relationships with others. Furthermore, it follows that mental health difficulties also need to be considered from this perspective (i.e. located within the social context). This view contrasts with an individualist approach that proposes people exist quite separately from one another and subsequently locates mental health difficulties solely within the individual.

Current thinking suggests that mental health difficulties can be traced to a combination of biological, social and psychological factors. In other words, it is thought that we all have genetic and biological vulnerabilities to particular problems but that this alone is not enough to trigger a mental health difficulty. In order for this to happen the added ingredient of social and psychological factors is also required. This includes where we live and work, our interpersonal experiences, our degree of connectedness with others and our social status. For example, Mr X may have an underlying vulnerability towards depression, but this may or may not occur depending on his life experiences. Experiences involving loss or trauma, such as bereavement, separation and divorce, redundancy, or even physical illness, are all potential triggers. Taking the latter as an example, if Mr X experiences a serious physical illness it is likely to affect many aspects of his life, including employment, social interaction and the ability to look after himself independently. These resulting social and psychological difficulties leave Mr X in a position where there is increased risk of his underlying vulnerability to depression being triggered.

If we overlook the social context when we are trying to understand and treat mental health problems, then we fail to address a fundamental part of these difficulties. In addition, it is likely that the social and interpersonal difficulties commonly experienced when mental health problems occur may be significantly compounded if we fail to take these factors into account. In turn, this may lead to further difficulties for the individual concerned and in many cases can end up resulting in a worse prognosis.

I have written this book for a wide range of people including those experiencing mental health problems and those who have a professional or personal interest. This latter group includes individuals working in the mental health profession and allied fields (i.e. education and general health), academics, researchers, students and those who are close to someone experiencing mental health difficulties. In addition, I hope that it will appeal to people who may not have any direct involvement with mental health but are curious to learn more. My wish is that by reading through these pages you will gain a richer understanding of mental health and in particular the important role that mutual support plays in psychological wellbeing.

The book has two main aims. The first is to impart information about the importance of the social context in understanding and treating mental health problems, with a specific focus on how vital mutual support is to our mental health. The second is to focus on the provision of mutual support and to give the reader practical information and suggestions as to how mutual support ideas may be applied. For example, I will provide advice with regard to accessing this type of support, with information provided about different services and groups both within and outside the UK. I will also discuss how to apply some of the ideas in the book to inform and benefit mental health practice. I conclude with some more general thoughts about how psychological wellbeing can be understood as a shared responsibility and how we can all benefit from learning about and practising a mutual support philosophy. Overall, I hope to provide an alternative way of thinking about and understanding mental health and to demonstrate that positive change is possible.

Part I of this book begins by defining what mutual support is and proceeds to describe its processes and functions. Chapter 1 provides an overview of the theoretical underpinnings of mutual support and ways that it can be of benefit, specifically with regard to mental health. Chapter 2 explores how mutual support can be understood from a developmental perspective, and then examines mutual support across the lifespan. In Chapter 3 these ideas are extended to investigate how mental health difficulties can impact on social functioning, as well as exploring ways in which cultural and environmental factors may affect our mental health.

Part II examines provision of mutual support within mental health services. Chapter 4 begins by defining formal and informal help, and explores how these two different types of helping can be utilised. The chapter describes how statutory mental health services tend to be configured in a way where the emphasis is on formal help, often with very little or no thought given to informal help. This is examined from the perspective of 'helper' and 'helped', and subsequent power differentials are explored. The following two chapters proceed to examine different types of mental health provision that utilise informal help, or mutual support. Chapter 5 focuses on group therapy. It starts by giving an overview of this approach and then proceeds to look at different types of therapeutic groups, including mutual support groups. The chapter also examines the curative factors that have been identified in group therapy. Chapter 6 outlines the work of therapeutic communities, tracing their history, outlining their influence and examining their current place within mental health provision.

Part III focuses on applications of mutual support and how it can be utilised to achieve better mental health. Chapter 7 details the evidence base for applied mutual support and how it benefits psychological wellbeing. Chapter 8 is concerned with putting mutual support theory into practice. The chapter is divided into two separate sections. The first section is for those who are seeking support for mental health problems; information and recommendations are provided with regard to finding appropriate and reputable sources of mutual support. The second section is for those interested in developing and facilitating mutual support interventions and for those working within the field of mental health looking to apply mutual support to their own practice. Guidance is presented as to how mutual support theory can be applied using a variety of different ideas and approaches. Finally, Chapter 9 discusses the future of mutual support. It reflects on the importance mutual support has on psychological wellbeing and how current service provision tends to ignore this by focusing on the individual alone. This narrow emphasis ignores an alternative route to recovery that can be both clinically valuable and cost-effective. It concludes that we can all utilise mutual support to achieve better mental health, both for ourselves and for those around us.

PART I

Processes and Functions of Mutual Support

CHAPTER 1

What Is Mutual Support?

This book challenges the way that mental health difficulties are traditionally thought about and treated. In the Western world there is a tendency to view such difficulties as pathological and being due to an individual 'flaw'. In my opinion this is analogous to looking at a 360 degree view through a fixed gyroscope. As we stare down the lens, the image we see comprises a fraction of the view before us; in other words we cannot see the 'whole picture'.

Within these pages I attempt to unlock the gyroscope in order for us to widen our field of vision. I am hoping that this will enable us to reach a better understanding of mental health problems and therefore be in a more advantageous position to alleviate some of the suffering connected with these experiences. In particular, widening our vision requires us to see the individual within their particular context. When we do this it becomes apparent that none of us exist in isolation but rather are a product of our connections and relationships with others and the world around us.

Life is a constant interaction, and this profoundly influences our thoughts, feelings and behaviours, both in the way we view others and ourselves. Central to this idea is the concept of mutual support. In the following pages I will attempt to describe what mutual support is and why it is so vital to us. I will also be putting forward the view that if we do not acknowledge the importance of the social context when dealing with mental health problems, then our attempts to understand and to alleviate these difficulties will be seriously flawed.

As with any journey into new territory we need to start by mapping some reference points; in this case we need to begin by defining what mutual support is. At first glance this seems a straightforward task; however, as with many things in life, it is not quite so simple. This is due to the many different ways that the concept of mutual support has been described and employed over the years, with a multitude of terms and definitions having been used to express the same ideas, and often used interchangeably. These include 'mutual support', 'peer support', 'mutual help', 'mutual aid', 'self-help', 'self-help group', 'mutual help group', 'mutual support group' and 'support group'. In addition, just to complicate matters further, identical terms are frequently defined differently in the literature.

In order to avoid similar confusion here, let me begin by clarifying and defining the terms that I shall be employing. I have chosen to use 'mutual support' and 'mutual support group' as I believe these best describe the types of interactions this book is concerned with. These contrast with the rather more individualistic 'self-help' or 'self-help group', as described by Humphreys and Rappaport (1994):

> Self-help groups are voluntary associations of persons who share some status that results in difficulties with which the group tries to deal... The term self-help group is inaccurate in some respects, because one important feature of groups is that people help each other. 'Self-help' does not capture the mutually supportive atmosphere of groups, suggesting instead an ethos of rugged individualism. The term *mutual help group* is thus used by many researchers because it captures the egalitarian and communal aspects of groups. (p.218)

I will also be differentiating 'mutual support group' from 'support group'. In the strict sense, the former term refers to groups where the members of the group are responsible for facilitating. Thus, all members of the group, including the facilitators, experience similar difficulties. In contrast, the latter term is used more widely and includes groups where members experience similar difficulties, but the group facilitators are usually mental health professionals, such as therapists. This is an important distinction, especially with regard to how professionals may change the atmosphere and process of the group (Toro *et al.* 1988).

So, how to define mutual support? There are many definitions including the original one made by Katz and Bender (1976):

> ...peers who have come together for mutual assistance in satisfying a common need, overcoming a common handicap or life-disrupting problem, and bringing about desired social and/or personal change.

The initiators and members of such groups perceive that their needs are not, or cannot be, met by or through existing social institutions. (p.9)

This definition is much cited in the literature and applies to a wide range of organisations and groups. However, mutual support can also involve two people rather than a group and the following alternative encompasses both possibilities: '...people sharing a similar problem, who meet regularly to exchange information and to give and receive psychological support' (Pistrang, Barker and Humphreys 2008, p.110). These definitions illustrate how mutual support is distinguished from the more general concept of social support. Whereas they both involve support within individuals' social networks, mutual support also includes the added dimension of people facing *similar difficulties*.

More about social support

Research exploring mutual support has grown out of the bedrock of the social support literature. The latter has grown exponentially since the publication in the mid 1970s of two highly influential reviews concerned with the impact of social relationships on physical and emotional wellbeing (Cassel 1976; Cobb 1976). Two decades later Cutrona (1996) estimated that there had been more than 4000 papers published on the subject.

As with mutual support, there are similar difficulties defining social support and there is still no widespread agreement. Taylor (2003) summarised past attempts at defining social support as:

Information from others that one is loved and cared for, esteemed and valued, and part of a network of communication and mutual obligations from parents, a spouse or lover, other relatives, friends, social and community contacts such as clubs, or even a devoted pet. (p.235)

Despite the conceptual difficulties, the body of research that has accumulated over the last three decades attests to the benefits of social support. A robust association between social support and physical and psychological wellbeing is now well established (Helgeson and Cohen 1996; Sarason, B.R., Sarason and Pierce 1990) and there is strong epidemiological evidence linking social support to lower risk for all-cause morbidity and mortality (House, Landis and Umberson 1988).

In contrast, it has generally been shown that poor social support is associated with poor mental health and physical health outcomes (Bloom 1990; Hogan, Linden and Najarian 2002).

Although it is generally proposed that social support *results* in increased psychological and physical wellbeing, we still know very little about the possible causal influence due to the largely correlational nature of the studies (Dooley 1985; Wortman and Dunkel-Schetter 1987). There is a diverse range of claims with regard to how social support may function to provide such benefits. Cohen and Wills (1985) put forward the 'stress-buffering hypothesis' suggesting that social support exerts a beneficial effect by influencing the individual's appraisals of potential stressors and coping resources. This links with Lazarus's transactional model of stress (Lazarus 1975), which proposes that a stress response is triggered when the individual appraises that they do not have sufficient resources to cope.

Whereas the two theories described above are based on the idea that social support is beneficial at times when stress is high, there are also claims that social support is beneficial even when stress levels are low. For example, the 'direct effects hypothesis' proposes that all social support is beneficial, whether or not there is perceived stress (Barrera 1986). Sarason, I.G. Sarason and Pierce (1990) expand this idea further by suggesting that benefits are derived from the *perception* that social support is available, whatever the actual reality is; this is described as 'perceived social support' (Dunkel-Schetter and Bennett 1990).

Supportive interactions

The findings from the social support literature have far-reaching implications, especially within the area of mental health. People suffering from mental health problems often experience difficulties interacting and connecting with others and may consequently become isolated, both from their peers and from wider society. This is taken up in Chapter 3 but before we explore these issues we first need to establish what constitutes a supportive interaction. However, it should also be borne in mind that classifying the properties of both social and mutual support is extremely problematic due to the complex and varied interactions that make up these phenomena.

Types of supportive interactions

To date, three main types of supportive interactions have been described. These are *informational, emotional* and *instrumental support* (Hogan *et al.* 2002).

Informational support includes the sharing of knowledge in order to provide advice and/or guidance and is thought to increase the recipient's coping skills and sense of mastery and control. In contrast, *emotional support* includes the expression of caring and concern as well as the communication of empathy. Emotional support is believed to reduce distress by enhancing self-esteem, decreasing feelings of isolation and stigma, and encouraging the expression of feelings. Last, *instrumental support* includes the provision of material goods and tangible resources to help solve practical tasks. This has been found to increase the recipient's sense of control by enabling them to do more.

The most beneficial type of support depends on individual context and needs. There is even evidence to suggest that support which does not match the individual's needs may be harmful (Cutrona 1990). It is thought that informational support is most beneficial when the stressor is relatively controllable, whereas emotional support is more helpful when the stressor is relatively uncontrollable (Helgeson and Gottlieb 2000). In addition, informational support is recognised as being more valuable if the provider is perceived as having experiential knowledge. This kind of knowledge is that gained from personal experience and is especially pertinent to mutual support, where individuals with similar problems join together to help one another. There are a number of theories as to why mutual support is beneficial to psychological wellbeing and these are outlined below.

Shared experience and understanding

Sharing experiences with other people who face a similar stressor is expected to lead to validation, normalisation of the experience, reduction in social and emotional isolation and a sense of belonging (Lieberman 1993). People facing a similar stressor are able to understand one another's situation in a way that naturally occurring social network members may not. There is evidence that in times of stress, natural social networks do not always behave in a supportive manner, partly from lack of understanding and partly from feelings of threat. For example, studies have shown that family members and friends of people who faced cancer, or people who had been victimised by a traumatic event such as rape, tend to discourage expression of feelings and instead try to distract the person from their problems. This is due to a belief that it could be harmful for the person to talk about the experience (Coates and Winston 1983; Dunkel-Schetter 1984; Peters-Golden 1982).

The helper-therapy principle

Riessman (1965) proposed that having opportunities to help others instils a feeling of self-efficacy and competence. In addition, the expectation is that peers will be able to provide sound advice and useful ideas about ways of coping because they have firsthand experience of the stressor. Empirical support for this principle has been provided by an observational behavioural measurement of the helping transactions that occur in mutual support groups for people with serious mental health problems, where giving help to others predicted psychosocial adjustment (Roberts et al. 1999).

The helper-therapy principle was extended by Maton (1988), in his bi-directional support hypothesis. This states that people who both provide and receive support will experience greater wellbeing than those involved in only one of these two processes. Group members who both gave and received support reported lower levels of depression, higher self-esteem and higher levels of satisfaction than those who predominantly gave or received support.

Social comparison theory

In times of uncertainty and stress, people compare themselves with others to evaluate their feelings and abilities (Festinger 1954). These *lateral comparisons* may normalise experiences as the individual learns that others suffer similar problems and share similar hopes, fears and concerns. There are also *upward* and *downward comparisons*. Helgeson and Mickelson (1995) observed that people engage in social comparison for reasons other than self-evaluation; self-improvement is typically accomplished by comparing oneself to someone who is perceived as better off. This person then acts as a role model, providing a source of inspiration to move forward. In contrast, downward comparisons refer to comparing oneself to someone perceived as worse off in order to feel better about one's own circumstances thus enhancing self-esteem.

Mutual support in the 21st century

Over the past three decades, the industrialised world has seen a steady increase in the number of people who turn to mutual support groups and organisations in order to help them cope during times of need (Jacobs and Goodman 1989; Kessler, Mickelson and Zhao 1997). Despite this, the majority of mental health services still continue to approach mental health difficulties from an individualistic stance and frequently give little thought to the wider social context and to mutual support. Some possible reasons for this will be explored in Chapter 4.

Returning to thinking about different types of supportive interactions, it is worth noting that mutual support groups generally offer informational and emotional support rather than instrumental (material) support. Does this mean that increased interest in mutual support groups is due to a decrease of informational and emotional support in our day-to-day lives? When we consider the societal changes that have occurred within the industrialised world over the last century or so this does tend to make sense. For example, whereas our material wealth has increased, many means of obtaining social support have diminished, including the breaking up of traditional family structures and communities. In our current climate it is not unusual for people to live alone, many miles from their families. In addition, many of us do not even know our neighbours, let alone those in the wider community.

This diminishment of our naturally occurring social support networks means that we now have to be much more proactive in seeking out social support and developing these networks ourselves. This is not always an easy task, and it becomes even more difficult when mental health problems are present. Chapter 3 discusses how mental health difficulties can affect social functioning and the ability to form mutually supportive relationships. Before exploring this we need to have an understanding of why mutual support is so important to us as human beings. The next chapter attempts to provide this by looking at mutual support from a developmental perspective.

CHAPTER 2

Mutual Support from a Developmental Perspective

A social species

The idea of mutual support being an essential element of what it means to be human is nothing new. Over 2000 years ago the Greek philosopher Aristotle defined man as a political animal and made the assertion that the individual cannot exist in social isolation. At the beginning of the last century, the Russian anarchist and theorist Peter Kropotkin described mutual support as the oldest form of help known to humanity. In his book *Mutual Aid: A Factor of Evolution* (1902/1972) he illustrates very convincingly that all living creatures depend on one another for survival. He proposed that mutual support and cooperation are fundamental human needs and furthermore are responsible for social progress.

Human beings are essentially a social species. We have a natural inclination to interact with and form connections with one another and have an innate propensity to organise ourselves into groups, whether this be at the level of family, community or nation. Indeed, from an evolutionary perspective we are social in nature. We are born related, and as we develop we continue to require relationships, both in order to survive and to reproduce successfully. In other words, we have an innate need to seek out and positively respond to close social ties (Barrett, Dunbar and Lycett 2001).

Human infants, unlike many other species, are born relatively helpless and remain dependent on caregivers for a significant period following birth in order to survive. Our early development is primarily a social process, with the family or group we are brought up in providing the principal social context within which this development occurs. Central to this is the attachment relationship we form with our primary caregiver. The study of attachment and its implications for continuing development was first studied by a British psychoanalyst named John Bowlby.

Attachment theory

Attachment theory (Bowlby 1969, 1973, 1980) forms a descriptive and explanatory framework concerned with understanding human attachments and relationships from infanthood across the lifespan. The first attachment relationship occurs in the first year of life and this forms the foundation from which we build all subsequent attachments and relationships.

Research has shown that during the first few months of life infants will orientate and signal without discriminating between people. This begins to change around the age of five to seven months, when they start to discriminate one or two preferred persons. The infant is more likely to smile at these people and be comforted by them. In the next phase, between seven and nine months of age, they will attempt to maintain proximity to these preferred persons. For example, they will follow them by crawling and become distressed if the person leaves – this often takes the form of screaming or crying. In addition, they start to become wary of unfamiliar persons. This latter phase is usually taken to signal the onset of attachment.

Following the formation of an attachment relationship, any temporary separation from the primary caregiver (usually the mother) will result in the following sequential emotional reactions as identified by Robertson and Bowlby (1952):

1. *Protest*, i.e. active searching, crying, resisting others' attempts at soothing.

2. *Despair*, i.e. passivity and sadness.

3. *Detachment*, i.e. actively disregarding and avoiding the caregiver when she returns (this is thought to be a type of defensive

behaviour, in other words it functions to defend against the pain of the separation).

Interestingly, very similar behaviour has been observed in primate infants when they are separated from their caregivers. This led Bowlby to propose that the infant–caregiver attachment is of evolutionary significance, arguing that it has developed to ensure the infant stays close to their caregiver, thus protecting them from danger.

Attachment style

A student of Bowlby named Mary Ainsworth was involved in testing and extending many of his ideas. In particular, she played a major role in suggesting that several attachment styles exist. Ainsworth and her colleagues developed a method called the 'Strange Situation' for assessing how well attached the infant/child is to their caregiver (Ainsworth *et al.* 1978). This consists of a number of episodes involving the infant being left by their caregiver for a period of time and then returning to them. It also includes a stranger entering the room where the infant and caregiver are, and remaining there when the caregiver leaves. The stranger stays with the infant for a while and then leaves too. The infant is thus left alone until the caregiver returns to them. Four different attachment types have been distinguished following observations of infants' behaviour during these episodes. Ainsworth *et al.* (1978) identified the first three styles, whilst Main and Solomon (1990) were responsible for identifying the fourth. These are:

- secure
- anxious/avoidant
- anxious/resistant
- disorganised.

SECURE ATTACHMENT STYLE

Typical behaviour of child – The child protests and is clearly distressed at the caregiver's departure. They are comforted by the caregiver's return and subsequently resume exploration of their environment, returning to the caregiver at times when they require reassurance. Thus the child uses the caregiver as a secure base.

Typical behaviour of caregiver – The caregiver responds to the child's emotional and physical needs in an appropriate, prompt and consistent manner.

ANXIOUS/AVOIDANT ATTACHMENT STYLE

Typical behaviour of child – When the caregiver leaves, the child shows little or no distress and continues to explore their surroundings as if nothing has happened. The child shows little or no visible response to the caregiver on their return.

Typical behaviour of caregiver – When the child is distressed, the caregiver shows little response. They typically discourage the child from crying and encourage independence and exploration.

ANXIOUS/RESISTANT ATTACHMENT STYLE

Typical behaviour of child – The child shows sadness when their caregiver leaves but also tends to react warmly to the stranger when they enter the room. When the caregiver returns, the child shows ambivalence as well as a reluctance to warm to them, and returns to play.

Typical behaviour of caregiver – The caregiver tends to behave towards the child in an inconsistent manner; sometimes acting appropriately and sometimes being neglectful.

DISORGANISED ATTACHMENT STYLE

Typical behaviour of child – The child shows a deficiency of any coherent coping strategy and typically behaves in a disorganised manner.

Typical behaviour of caregiver – The caregiver typically exhibits frightening and disorientating behaviour. For example, there tends to be a fluctuation between intrusiveness, withdrawal and negativity. In addition there is often role and boundary confusion that may lead to child maltreatment such as physical and/or sexual abuse.

These four different attachment styles derive from the ways in which the caregiver and the child relate to one another. It is important to consider that this involves an *interaction* and a *reciprocal* exchange. This means that attachment style is determined by both the caregiver's *and* the child's behaviour. For example, the development of a secure attachment relationship and style depends to a large extent on the capacity of the caregiver to provide the child with a secure base, thus enabling the child to explore their environment safely. The caregiver provides an essential role in helping the child to make sense of the world, as well as enabling them to develop a sense of self in relation to other people. However, the way that the caregiver behaves towards the child is also influenced by the child's behaviour towards them. In addition, it is important to note that the caregiver's behaviour is influenced by the relationship that they had with their own caregiver, and by their own attachment style arising from this. Thus it is clear how previous generations shape future ones, and how intergenerational patterns emerge.

Clearly, the caregiver is unable to be with the child constantly and there will be periods when separation is unavoidable. The child gradually adapts to this experience, and the formation of a goal-corrected partnership begins. This is when the child begins to accommodate to their caregiver's needs; for example being prepared to wait alone if requested, until their caregiver returns. This development happens around the second to third year of age. There are further developments when the child starts to spend more time away from their caregiver; typically from school-age and beyond. Attachment relationships start to become less dependent on the concrete notion of physical proximity and more dependent on the abstract qualities of the relationship, such as trust and affection.

Bowlby proposed that, within early attachment relationships, the infant must form a sense of themselves in relation to others. Over time, this develops into an internal working model (IWM) of social relating. The IWM consists of learnt expectations relating to the responsiveness of the caregiver. Another way of understanding this is the idea of there being an internal representation of the attachment relationship, comprising a cognitive framework or structure where memories of the relationship are stored. This IWM subsequently generalises to new situations and people. In other words, it acts as a guide for future social interactions and helps inform an understanding of others with whom relationships are formed over the course of one's life.

Attachment across the lifespan

Bowlby believed that attachment theory could be applied across the lifespan and was not just something that influences behaviour during infancy and childhood: '…attachment behaviour [characterizes] human beings from the cradle to the grave' (Bowlby 1979, p.129). Indeed, attachment theory has now been applied to a variety of social behaviours across the lifespan including peer relationships; care-seeking by both children and adults (i.e. when sick or elderly); sexual attraction; intimate relationships; marital satisfaction and parenting.

Bowlby proceeded to explore the processes by which affectional bonds are forged and broken in order to further his understanding in this respect. These findings can be found in his trilogy where he explored attachment, separation and loss (Bowlby 1969, 1973, 1980). In the second volume he summarised attachment theory in three propositions:

> The first [proposition] is that when an individual is confident that an attachment figure will be available to him whenever he desires it, that person will be much less prone to either intense or chronic fear than will an individual who for any reason has no such confidence. The second proposition concerns the sensitive period during which such confidence develops. It postulates that confidence in the availability of attachment figures, or lack of it, is built up slowly during the years of immaturity – infancy, childhood, and adolescence – and that whatever expectations are developed during those years tend to persist relatively unchanged throughout the rest of life. The third proposition concerns the role of actual experience. It postulates that the varied expectations of the accessibility and responsiveness of attachment figures that individuals develop during the years of immaturity are tolerably accurate reflections of the experiences those individuals have actually had. (Bowlby 1973, p.235)

Bowlby originally thought that there was a *critical* period of infant development and that missing crucial experiences around this time was likely to adversely affect social development later on. He subsequently modified this and instead proposed that there was more likely to be a *sensitive* period for the development of secure attachments. For example, children who have poor early experiences, but who then proceed to have positive experiences later on, may also develop the capacity to make secure attachments.

It is important to pick up on Bowlby's theory that once attachment style has developed, it subsequently remains relatively unchanged throughout life. This hypothesis forms a fundamental part of Bowlby's work and it has been incredibly influential. The implications of such a hypothesis are far-reaching, as it proposes that our early relationships cast us in a particular way, which then influences all our subsequent relationships with others. This idea remains controversial, and current thinking suggests that representations of early relationships do not necessarily predict subsequent relationship outcomes in either a simple or straightforward fashion.

Although there is a bias towards continuity (due to IWMs acting rather like a filter through which new experiences are interpreted), there is also ample opportunity for change due to the numerous factors that might intervene to alter this. For example, it is likely that representations tend to be modified continuously as the individual experiences different types of attachment relationships across the lifespan (Carlson, Sroufe and Egeland 2004). In other words, our past does not unalterably determine our future relationships. Instead it would appear that the latter are determined by the history of attachment relationships in conjunction with current relationships and social contexts.

Findings to date suggest that social development involves continual construction, revision and integration of IWMs. For example, the negative impact of early attachment difficulties can be modified by subsequent experiences of mutually supportive relationships. This idea is consistent with the possibility of change based on the individual taking in new information and experiences.

Social relationships and personal identity

Bowlby proposed that the way we view ourselves (i.e. the mental model we hold of ourself) is dependent upon and in some way constituted by relationships with others. Bowlby put forward the idea that this begins in our experiences of early relationships with attachment figures:

> Confidence that an attachment figure is, apart from being accessible, likely to be responsive can be seen to turn on at least two variables: (a) whether or not the attachment figure is judged to be the sort of person who in general responds to calls for support and protection; [and] (b) whether or not the self is judged to be the sort of person towards whom anyone, and the attachment figure in particular, is likely to respond in a helpful way. Logically these variables are independent. In practice they are apt to be confounded. As a result, the model of the attachment figure and the model of the self are likely to develop so as to be complementary and mutually confirming. (Bowlby 1973, p.238)

The point that Bowlby makes can be illustrated by thinking about the development of a secure attachment style. Secure attachment correlates with the child having a model of their caregiver and key others being predictable, validating and responsive. As a result, they are more likely to have developed an internal working model of self as being worthy of help and of others being willing to help. They are also more likely to feel valued and understood and will subsequently possess a greater sense of security, increased self-esteem and confidence, a more optimistic view of social relationships and thus more effective strategies for getting help when needed.

Bowlby proposed that IWMs of attachment consist of two variables; the *model of other* and the *model of self.* The model of other relates to the degree that others are generally expected to be available and supportive whilst the model of self represents the degree to which the individual has been able to *internalise* a sense of self-worth. Bowlby suggested that these models develop within the individual in relation to each other, and that this usually happens in a complementary manner. For example, if the caregiver is sensitive and responsive to the needs of the child, then the child is more likely to develop a positive model of both self and other. However, there is also evidence to suggest that they can sometimes vary independently of each other; that is, a negative model of other and positive model of self, or vice versa (Bartholomew and Horowitz 1991).

Attachment and mental health

When Bowlby first started exploring attachment he was interested in trying to understand whether there was a connection between poor social relationships and psychopathology. As we have seen, Bowlby's model of attachment states that the development of the attachment relationship is a key developmental task that influences the child's representations of self and others. Bowlby further proposed that if the child develops a negative representation of self and others, they become more vulnerable to developing mental health problems.

Since Bowlby first made a connection between attachment and mental health, there have been numerous studies exploring this. It is now established that early attachment relationships form a very important foundation, both to individual development and to mental health. For example, research suggests that the loss of a parent in childhood is linked to an elevated risk of depression and various types of mental health difficulties in adulthood (Dietrich 2006; Lloyd 1980; Mäkikyrö et al. 1998). In addition, we now know that an association exists between insecure attachment and different forms of mental health problems

(Dozier, Stovall and Albus 1999). Conversely, a secure attachment style correlates with being more resilient and less prone to mental health problems.

The influence and importance of our social experiences, from the moment we are born and onwards, cannot be overemphasised. Social relationships influence how we view ourselves, how we feel and how we interact with others and the world around us. It follows that these experiences need to be included when we are thinking about and exploring mental health problems. Indeed, findings show that the main presenting problems of adults seeking psychological support are relationship and/or interpersonal difficulties and the subsequent distress caused (Horowitz 1979).

The perspective I take is that, in order to adequately address mental health problems it is necessary to have an understanding of an individual's social context (i.e. their life stage, connectedness and relationships with others, social standing, etc.). In other words, I do not believe that it is possible for mental health difficulties to be properly assessed and treated without these factors being taken into consideration. The next chapter picks up on this idea by exploring mental health from a social and interpersonal perspective. It begins by examining the correlation between mental health problems and difficulties in social functioning, and then considers the impact of environmental and cultural factors.

CHAPTER 3

Mental Health Difficulties and Social Functioning

As stated in the Introduction, current thinking suggests that mental health difficulties can be traced to a combination of biological, social and psychological factors. It is thought that we each have vulnerabilities to different difficulties and that this is where the idea of psychosocial factors is important to consider. For example, even if an individual has a biological vulnerability to depression, this may or may not develop depending on their life circumstances. If events occur that affect the capacity to function in day-to-day life (e.g. bereavement or physical illness that results in withdrawal from daily life), then this may trigger a depressive episode.

Taking the social and psychological context into consideration is vital in the understanding and treatment of mental health problems. This is essentially a socio-political perspective as it takes the view that in order to reach an informed understanding of any individual, there must be an understanding of the relation of that individual to others around them. Underlying this perspective is the belief that a person's identity is both dependent upon and in some way constituted by their relationships with others. This connects with the ideas talked about in the previous chapter where we looked at how interactions and relationships shape the way we view ourselves.

Difficulties in social functioning are frequently present when mental health problems are experienced. In other words, there is a correlation between mental health problems and difficulties in social functioning. These two factors form a complex cycle and can clearly end up compounding one another. For example, mental health problems can have a significant negative impact on the ability to interact socially and to form and sustain social relationships. Social isolation causes and exacerbates mental distress, and in turn the social exclusion and stigma associated with mental health compounds this isolation.

In many cases, experiencing mental health problems can result in exclusion from important areas of daily life. For example, employment is one such area that has significant implications for the individual, both with regard to social functioning and material factors. In addition, there is a strong correlation between mental health problems and homelessness, poverty and incarceration. Again it is not hard to see the connection between these factors and how difficulties in any one of these areas is going to increase the likelihood of the other factors occurring. Sadly, we live in a society where mental health problems continue to be stigmatised, and the result is that many people suffering these difficulties end up in an isolated and disempowered position.

In 2004 the UK mental health charity Mind conducted a national survey on social isolation and found that 84 per cent of people experiencing mental health problems reported feeling isolated, as opposed to 29 per cent of the general public. In addition, social isolation significantly impacts on the ability of those with mental health problems to cope with these difficulties and work towards recovery, as well as increasing the risk of suicide (Mind 2004).

Psychosocial stages and mental health

Mental health problems can strike at any age and the impact on the person affected can vary according to a number of factors. These include type of difficulties, individual circumstances and what is known as 'developmental stage'. In psychology, 'stage theories' refer to theories of development that characterise growth as a progression through a sequence of stages. One of the pioneers of psychological lifespan development was Erik Erikson, a developmental psychologist and psychoanalyst. Erikson's stage theory of psychosocial development (1968) is outlined in Table 3.1.

Erikson rejected Freud's view that all mental health difficulties can be traced to early childhood experiences and instead emphasised the influence of social factors throughout the life course. Erikson proposed that, as we proceed through life, we face particular experiences connected to different life stages resulting in various psychosocial crises that need to be worked through. Each crisis involves a relatively long period of time and may involve many years where the individual struggles to attain some degree of psychological strength. It is important to note that Erikson proposed the difficulties in each crisis are always there to some degree and may need to be reconfronted at different periods throughout life.

Table 3.1 Erikson's Psychosocial Stages of Personality Development (Erikson 1968)

Life stage	Psychosocial crisis	Developmental focus	Outcome
Infancy (Birth–18 mths)	Basic trust vs. basic mistrust	Trust in others	Security or mistrust
Early childhood (2–3 years)	Autonomy vs. shame and doubt	Personal control	Self-confidence or self-doubt
Preschool (3–5 years)	Initiative vs. guilt	Asserting control	Capable and able or lacking initiative
School age (6–11 years)	Industry vs. inferiority	Testing abilities	Competence or doubt of ability
Adolescence (12–18 years)	Identity vs. role confusion	Exploring independence	Strong sense of self or insecurity
Young adulthood (19–40 years)	Intimacy vs. isolation	Personal relationships	Secure relationships or not
Middle adulthood (40–65 years)	Generativity vs. stagnation	Career and family	Contribution or uninvolvement
Maturity (65+)	Ego integrity vs. despair	Reflection	Wisdom or regret/despair

Table 3.1 details eight life stages from infancy through to maturity, and the various psychosocial crises connected to each. For example, during adolescence there is a focus on becoming more independent as we

move towards adulthood. The outcome of this life stage is a clearer sense of self or, conversely, insecurity and confusion about our identity. The former is likely to result in a smoother transition to the next stage (i.e. young adulthood), whilst the latter results in more of a struggle. In the case of the latter, this insecurity and confusion, coupled with predisposing factors, may increase the likelihood of developing mental health difficulties.

In many cases mental health problems arise during adolescence and early adulthood. Developmentally, this is a crucial period involving the forming of friendships and intimate relationships, as well as establishing a coherent adult identity and sense of self. Taking this into consideration, it is not surprising that many individuals who experience mental health problems at this life stage frequently become socially and emotionally isolated. Subsequently, it can be extremely difficult to re-engage, with others and with life generally, and this can have considerable effects on self-esteem, confidence and the ability to participate in the world. It is easy to see how a vicious cycle can ensue in these circumstances, with the individual's social difficulties both compounding and perpetuating their mental health problems.

More generally, when people at any life stage experience mental health difficulties, their capacity for seeking out and maintaining relationships can be adversely affected, an effect that tends to increase with the seriousness of the mental health problem. Lyons, Perotta and Hancher-Kvam (1988) point out that social support networks are very often restricted for people experiencing serious mental health problems. Despite this, it would appear that these difficulties are frequently overlooked, or not given adequate attention, in most mental health services. For example, the focus of the majority of mental health services is primarily on formal help (i.e. help provided by professionals) and there is often very little thought given to peer support and the importance of the social context. This is explored further in the next chapter.

Although I accept that, for many people, professional support is both helpful and necessary, I also believe more thought needs to be given to ways that people experiencing mental health difficulties can help one another. The problem with offering formal support alone, especially to those with longer-term mental health difficulties, is that there is a risk of compounding feelings of dependency. Furthermore, there are issues connected to disempowerment and learnt helplessness, as the person being helped is placed in a position where they have no opportunity to reciprocate. This can further intensify feelings of having nothing of value to offer and is likely to reduce self-esteem and undermine confidence to an even greater extent.

The socio-political context: Why we need mutual support more than ever

As mentioned in Chapter 1, traditional support networks are rapidly diminishing in the Western world due to a combination of expanding levels of industrialisation and urbanisation that can be traced back to the Industrial Revolution. These developments have resulted in major societal shifts including increased movement at an individual level. As a consequence it is no longer the norm for people to stay in one area and to live in a community comprising family members and close neighbours. Instead, communities have dispersed and many people now live miles away from the families and the people they grew up with. This has resulted in increasing numbers of people living alone, often with few contacts in the area where they reside. Although we still talk about 'communities', the reality is that residential areas are frequently made up of people who are strangers to one another.

As well as the social shifts brought about through factors such as increased industrialisation and urbanisation there are also enforced shifts that occur due to more sinister reasons, such as political tension, war or natural disaster. In these cases the individual usually has no choice, and social networks are forcibly broken up. People caught up in these experiences have to deal with the added complexity of trauma, loss and dislocation, often with devastating consequences.

One thing is clear, whether people choose to move to seek better opportunities in the form of education, employment and greater financial reward, or whether they are forced to move due to situations outside of their control, in each case there is usually an emotional cost. Many of us now reside in areas where we have very little connection with the people around us. This is especially so in cities, where acknowledging or speaking to people we do not know is generally seen as suspicious, and in some cases, downright perverse. Everything appears geared up to be done as quickly as possible with the least amount of social interaction possible. We consequently function in a world where alienation and paranoia are frequently experienced and have increasingly become part of the way we respond to and interact with each other. Do we not feel an initial suspicion when a stranger smiles at us, nods a hello or offers to help us with our heavy bags when we are trying to negotiate a flight of stairs? Taking all of this into consideration, is it any wonder that mental health problems are so prevalent in modern society? And is it really surprising that those who suffer mental health problems experience such difficulties in coping and working towards recovery in such environments?

Current prevalence of mental health problems

So, how common are mental health problems? Estimates vary, but the World Health Organization (WHO) reports that one in four people will experience mental health problems at some stage in their lifetime (WHO 2001).

Despite these high frequencies, people who experience such difficulties remain one of the most socially excluded groups. They are frequently denied the same rights to employment, housing, education and community participation as the rest of the population. Evidence suggests that this discrimination is found within many different areas including general practitioner (GP) practices, medical services, banks and insurance companies. In fact, mental health discrimination is such a big problem that a number of government and media initiatives have been set up to try to tackle these concerns. Interestingly, research shows that contact with those suffering from mental health problems tends to reduce negative stereotypes (Corrigan and Penn 1999). This supports the theory that efforts need to be focused on social integration and equal opportunities for those who are experiencing, or have experienced, mental health problems.

The influence of the social environment

There is evidence that the type of social environment we live in has a significant effect on our mental health. For example, research suggests urban environments have a pathogenic influence. Being born or brought up in a city increases the risk of schizophrenia; in fact the risk of developing schizophrenia is up to three times higher for urban residents than those living in rural areas. Similarly, first onset cases of schizophrenia are concentrated in the socially deprived areas of cities. Why should this be? Is there some connection with the social factors operating within these environments, such as those described above?

In the 1970s two independent large-scale studies compared the course and outcome of individuals diagnosed with schizophrenia in developing and developed countries (Sartorius, Jablensky and Shapiro 1977; Waxler 1979). They found that those residing in developing countries had a better prognosis. The reasons for these findings have been disputed for decades and there is still no definitive answer. However, various studies exploring schizophrenia in different cultural settings and ethnic minority groups have suggested several possibilities. Two landmark studies conducted by the WHO (Jablensky *et al.* 1992; WHO 1979) indicate that strong social networks and cultural attitudes play a significant role. For example, in developing countries, recovery from severe mental health problems is more common. It is thought that this is connected to the strong familial and community networks that are still the norm within these countries, as well as the fact that people with severe mental health problems often continue to be engaged in occupational activities. In contrast, the majority of individuals living in industrialised countries no longer experience such extended social and community support systems and are frequently prevented from working for a number of different reasons. It is noteworthy that severe mental health problems tend towards a chronic course for these individuals.

These findings provide further insight into the ways that social relationships and interactions connect to our self-identity and to our mental health. For example, if those experiencing mental health problems are viewed as being unable to contribute to society, through working or through taking on particular responsibilities, then this is going to have a strong negative influence on the way they view themselves and their capabilities. It is clear how this can result in a negative feedback loop where mental health difficulties are reinforced and perpetuated through lack of opportunities for social participation and self-development. As Skilton (2007) states:

> Psychiatric disorders and suicidal attempts were more likely to occur in people facing socio-economic disadvantage: that is people with unskilled occupations or who were unemployed, who lacked formal qualifications, who were renting accommodation from a local authority or housing association, who were living alone, or were separated or divorced. (p32)

Although there have been many improvements in the way that mental health problems are understood and treated, we still have a way to go before we can say that we live in a society that is accepting and tolerant of these experiences. Bearing this in mind, we also need to think about the major shift that has occurred within mental health treatment in the UK since the 1990's with the advent of 'Care in the Community'. This government initiative was introduced with the intention of moving people with mental health problems out of hospital settings into the 'community'.

Care in the Community

Since the introduction of Care in the Community, increasing numbers of inpatient services have been and continue to be closed, with funding channelled into alternative types of community-based care. The phrase itself is suggestive of an inclusive community that cares. However, in reality few communities exist, especially within inner-city areas, and those that do are not always welcoming of people who are experiencing mental health problems. This is evidenced earlier in the chapter when we discussed the continued stigma and discrimination that surrounds mental health. However, this tends to be overlooked or ignored. The upshot is that increasing numbers of individuals experiencing mental health problems now reside in the 'community', whilst the 'community' continues to demonstrate all manner of discrimination against them.

In my clinical work within an inner-London acute mental health inpatient service, I bear witness to many stories that pay testament to the struggle with life outside hospital. The stories are different but the themes are similar; exclusion, discrimination, stigma and social isolation predominate. Like most other inpatient mental health units across the UK, the service I work in operates a short-term treatment policy. However, a significant number of those discharged are re-admitted within a relatively short space of time, and this pattern tends to repeat for many of these people. This phenomenon is known as 'the revolving door'. Although these individuals are not kept in hospital long-term (as was the case in the past), in many ways they remain in this position, albeit with breaks when they are discharged.

When we consider the reality that most people are being discharged to, we start to get a clearer picture of why this revolving door exists. The majority of those admitted do not have their own accommodation and are usually discharged to a rehabilitation service, a supported project or a homeless person's hostel. These options are all short-stay (from a few months to a maximum of two years), after which there will be an expectation to move on to another step-down project, and so on. Similarly most day services have now been reconfigured to operate short-stay policies. The result is that many people with severe and enduring mental health problems are constantly moved from one place to another, often at the point when they are just starting to feel comfortable in their environment and form relationships with those around them. When we consider that many of these individuals already struggle with social interaction and relationships, this is clearly not a helpful model. Factor in the discrimination and stigma connected to mental health problems and it is not surprising that many individuals with these difficulties end up in a revolving door scenario.

An important aim of inpatient care is to offer asylum in the original sense of the word (i.e. shelter or protection from danger). This danger can take many forms and in many cases the 'community' can be the cause of this fear. To address these concerns, mental health provision needs to offer the individual support and safety, but also needs to explore how the experience of feeling supported and safe can continue in the longer term and eventually be internalised. This requires being mindful of the individual *and* their social context. Instead, the irony is that services set up to address mental health problems are in many ways mirroring and repeating the same societal dynamics that perpetuate these difficulties; that is, pathologising the individual and avoiding any prolonged contact. This will be examined further in Part II, which explores mental health provision in more depth. It starts by detailing how services tend to be configured with an emphasis on formal help, and then outlines alternative approaches that utilise mutual, or informal, support as part of the therapeutic endeavour.

PART II

Mutual Support and Mental Health Provision

CHAPTER 4

Formal and Informal Help

In the Western world we have cultivated a belief that knowledge about mental health resides with professionals alone, and that difficulties can only be treated through the professional sharing this information. However, individuals who experience mental health problems also hold vital knowledge and expertise; they live with these difficulties and have often acquired valuable information about different ways to cope. This experiential knowledge is an incredibly important resource, both for the individual and for others. When it is shared with others who are in a similar position it is known as 'informal help'; described as '…helping between ordinary people in everyday settings' (Barker and Pistrang 2002, p.362). Informal help can be differentiated from 'formal help' provided by trained professional helpers such as mental health professionals.

Help-seeking behaviour

Help-seeking behaviour refers to what people do when they perceive that they need support from others. Overall, studies exploring help-seeking behaviour in people facing mental health difficulties indicate a general preference for informal over formal help (Barker *et al.* 1990). It has been proposed that people's help-seeking behaviour may be conceptualised as a pathway, where minor problems are taken to informal helpers, more persistent problems are handled by non-specialist helpers, such as general practitioners, and severe difficulties are dealt with by mental health specialists (Barker and Pistrang 2002). This has been likened to people employing their own form of 'stepped care', beginning with the most accessible, community-based forms of support and only progressing to professional help if their difficulties are not resolved satisfactorily (Haaga 2000).

A number of possible reasons as to why people generally prefer to seek out informal rather than formal help have been proposed. These include services being located too far away, costing too much or not fitting with individual needs. However, even if these obstacles are absent, it is generally found that people still prefer to talk with trusted individuals from their social networks – '…people who are willing to listen when they are ready to talk' (Cowen 1982, p.385).

In line with this, Goldberg and Huxley (1992) concluded that, although 'episodes of disorder are fairly common in the population… only a small minority will be seen by mental health professionals' (p.5). They estimated that, of the 300 people out of 1000 who experience mental health problems every year in Great Britain:

- 230 will visit a GP

- 102 of these will then be diagnosed as having a mental health problem

- 24 of these will be then referred to a specialist psychiatric service

- 6 will then become inpatients in psychiatric hospitals.

The UK National Survey of Psychiatric Morbidity found that less than 14 per cent of people with a non-psychotic disorder were receiving any kind of professional treatment (Bebbington et al. 2000). The World Health Organization (WHO 2001) predicted that up to two thirds of people suffering mental health problems never seek help because of the associated discrimination and stigma.

Even when individuals are receiving support from formal sources, evidence shows that they also tend to engage in seeking out informal support. For example, Cross, Sheehan and Kahn (1980) found that participants in both treatment and control groups in a comparative therapy outcome study sought out informal help. In fact, the rate of informal help-seeking was greater in the two treatment groups than in the control group (the control group received no formal therapy). This may provide an alternative explanation for some of the gains reported by the therapy groups compared to the control group in that the former were receiving a combination of formal *and* informal help. These findings are not so surprising when we consider that formal help such as therapy would be expected to help the individual access and discuss their thoughts and feelings more easily. In turn it may be more likely that these experiences would then be shared with others outside of the therapy.

Within mental health care services there is a tendency for formal and informal help to be perceived in a rather dichotomous way, instead of seeing them as mutually beneficial. For example, healthcare professionals frequently appear quite reluctant to accept experiential knowledge and informal help as legitimate sources of knowledge and support. In addition, they can tend to view informal help as a threat to professional expertise. As a result there are often few opportunities for mental health service users to share experiences with peers and to learn from each other in any formally structured settings within services.

'Helper' and 'helped'

The majority of statutory mental health services are configured in a way that comprises mental health professionals delivering care and treatment to those who are experiencing difficulties. This essentially involves a structure where there is a delineated split between 'helper' and 'helped' and a resulting power differential where those responsible for the treatment of mental health difficulties are placed in a position of authority and control. The latter increases incrementally in response to the seriousness of the mental health problem. So, for example, those who are perceived as suffering from difficulties to a degree that they are believed to require hospitalisation can end up being legally sectioned if they do not consent to this treatment. This removes the individual's right to choose whether or not they wish to receive treatment as they are judged to lack insight into the nature and degree of their difficulties. In these situations the power differential is at its most extreme as the mental health professional has the power to treat the individual, even if that individual objects. It is fair to say that this is a complex area where there are no easy answers and each case must be assessed accordingly.

Within this paradigm is the perception that the mental health difficulty resides solely within the individual and should be treated as such. For example, mental health problems are treated as 'symptoms' emanating from and located within the individual, and the individual is thus placed in the position of 'helped'. In many ways this can be viewed as defensive behaviour functioning to contain the difficulties within the individual alone and thus keep the 'helped' in a separate and distinct position to those who are perceived to be 'well'. As stated earlier, this approach is commonly employed in mental health care but at what cost to those being helped by these services?

The experience of suffering mental health difficulties is, in itself, enough to provoke feelings of helplessness. This is especially relevant when the individual has a long history of mental health difficulties. Mental health service users frequently report feeling ostracised and alienated due to the nature of their difficulties. In addition, they often feel that they do not have anything valuable to offer. Long-term mental health problems can result in a situation where the individual concerned is continually experiencing being on the receiving end of being helped in various ways. If there is no counterbalance to this, for example by providing experiences where the individual's own sense of agency is addressed, it can result in the individual feeling they have no internal resources that are of any value. This ends up in a dynamic where a vicious cycle ensues: the more help the individual receives from professionals, the more dependent they become and the more helpless they feel. I suggest that this vicious cycle is further compounded by the power imbalance that traditionally exists within mental health services.

When we look at the approach embodied within current mental health provision it is difficult to believe its foundations are embedded in one where mutual support was recognised as central to recovery. I will now attempt to outline this history and explain how mutual support was supplanted by a very different approach to understanding and treating mental health difficulties.

Tracing mutual support – history of mental health provision in the UK

During the 18th century, society dramatically changed the way it treated those who were deemed mentally ill. This happened against the backdrop of massive social change connected to the beginnings of the modern industrial age. Up until the mid-18th century there was only one hospital in the UK for those with mental health problems, the Bethlem Hospital. Founded in 1247, the Bethlem started to admit people with mental health problems in the mid-14th century and was infamous for its brutality. As a result of the scarcity of resources, the majority of individuals experiencing mental health problems struggled as best they could in the community; either living with their families or ending up in a custodial institution such as the poorhouse, workhouse or gaol.

Towards the middle of the 18th century, the introduction of the Vagrancy Act gave the state power to lock up those who were deemed to suffer from 'lunacy' for as long as these symptoms continued, and individuals were often kept chained to the wall. This heralded the beginnings of a movement to incarcerate those with mental health problems and the idea of segregating these individuals from the rest of society gathered momentum. Private provision in the form of 'madhouses' began to take root where 'care' usually involved barbaric practice and cruel punishments. In addition, there was little incentive to improve the lives of those held there, as most of these institutions were run for profit and little else. During this era there was little understanding of mental health and those experiencing such difficulties were frequently viewed as both morally inferior and 'untreatable'.

Moral treatment and The York Retreat

Towards the end of the 18th century mental health treatment took a dramatic turn. This largely came about due to the unexpected and mysterious death of a Quaker named Hannah Mills whilst she was a patient in the York Asylum. The Quaker community were so shocked by this event that they decided to found their own establishment for fellow Quakers suffering from what was then known as 'the loss of reason'.

The York Retreat opened in 1796 under the guidance and charge of William Tuke, a Quaker tea and coffee merchant. It pioneered humane treatment; aiming to recognise and nurture the intact part of the patient's personality through providing an environment where patients became part of a large family-like unit. The emphasis was on building kind and mutually respectful relationships against the backdrop of pleasant, quiet surroundings. Patients were free to wander within the grounds and there was also an expectation to engage in meaningful activities, such as helping with tasks connected to the running of the establishment.

This approach came to be known as 'moral treatment' – Samuel Tuke (William's grandson) borrowed this phrase from the French physician Phillipe Pinel when describing the methods of The York Retreat in a book published in 1813 called *Description of the Retreat*. For 25 years following its publication, this book was regarded as the standard British text on mental health care and treatment. This gives an indication of the importance of these ideas at this time.

Kennard (2000) describes moral treatment of mental health problems by considering its ideology, practice and principles.

The ideology behind moral treatment is concerned with ideas about how society needs to be organised, as well as the consequences of this for the individuals who make up that society. So, for example, during the 18th century, those suffering mental health problems were seen as morally inferior, treated inhumanely and thought to be beyond help. Moral treatment challenged this by arguing that those experiencing mental health problems were morally equal to others and should be treated as such.

The practice of moral treatment involved the application of humane principles within a mutually respectful and supportive social setting. Connected to this was the expectation that individuals with mental health problems should be engaged in the everyday tasks of the community in order to provide a sense of routine, purpose and achievement.

Last, the principles underlying this approach include the belief that mental health problems are 'curable' and that the social environment is a fundamental factor in achieving this aim. This can be illustrated by considering the impact of social expectations. For example, if someone experiencing mental health problems is perceived and treated as being incapable of engaging in meaningful activity, then they are eventually likely to believe this themselves. The expectation of patients at The York Retreat was that they were both rational and responsible.

The ethos of The York Retreat stood in sharp contrast to the inhumane and frequently barbaric practices employed in 18th century madhouses. In the latter, conditions were frequently squalid, and punishment, restrictions and enforced idleness usually prevailed. The York Retreat also differed from these 'madhouses' in that the mental health of the individuals who became patients there actually started to improve. News of this success spread far and wide, leading to numerous debates about mental health provision. By the mid-18th century Parliament passed a series of laws, known as the 1845 Lunacy Act. This required every county in England and Wales to provide a purpose-built asylum for people suffering mental health problems. It also consolidated a shift away from parochial, privatised approaches to a state-run custodial approach that segregated those experiencing mental health problems from the general population.

The decline of moral treatment

On the one hand, this was a time of great excitement and hope. The York Retreat had created a revolution in humane treatment for those with mental health problems. It was also responsible for pioneering the idea that mental health problems could improve and so changed the task of the mental health institution from a place of custody to that of rehabilitation. However, somewhat ironically, by the time the last county asylums were being built in the 1890s, moral treatment had largely disappeared.

Kennard (2000) proposes a number of reasons for the decline of moral treatment. First there is a sense that moral treatment was killed by its own success. Social reformers were very excited by The York Retreat's achievements and persuaded both the English Parliament and the American States to provide similar institutions. However, these were built on a significantly larger scale, and the upshot was that the aim of establishing a community atmosphere was no longer adhered to. Second, in 1890 another series of laws was introduced, known as the 1890 Lunacy Act, which stated that only the most incurable should be admitted to hospital – as a result institutions took on a more custodial role. Last, the individuals who founded The York Retreat were reluctant to establish a new profession of experts in moral treatment.

It should be remembered that The Retreat was developed as an alternative to the madhouses, where the medical profession claimed to be experts in the treatment of those patients such as the unfortunate Hannah Mills. In contrast, the ethos at The Retreat was to treat patients with respect and to provide opportunities for social interaction and engagement in everyday tasks and activities. The pioneers of this approach reasoned that this could be practised by anyone with the ability to apply humanity and common sense. An 'expert' role was in many respects diametrically opposed to the very ideas they stood for, and they therefore declined to take up this position. If they had, standard mental health provision may have progressed very differently to the way it has.

The birth of psychiatry and medical dominance

Compared to the pioneers of moral treatment, the fledgling psychiatrists were not so modest. In contrast they were very keen to establish themselves as a reputable profession and proposed that medicine would be the 'cure' for mental health problems. Linked to this, they were eager to gain control of the asylum system and to construct a credible knowledge base to underpin a form of medical authority over mental health problems. It followed that the medical profession's claims to be the natural authority responsible for those with mental health problems went unchallenged. By the end of the 19th century different researchers proposed various taxonomies of mental 'disorders', and medical dominance was established.

Although The Retreat continued, and indeed continues to this day, it was not until the early 20th century that other similarly structured organisations started to emerge in the form of planned environment therapy and therapeutic communities. It is interesting to note that the therapeutic community approach really took hold within certain periods during the last century, just as The Retreat had done. But similarly to The Retreat this popularity was short-lived and an individual-centric, symptom-focused approach once again became dominant. This is likely to be connected to changes in the way mental health services are delivered, such as the purchaser–provider split within the National Health Service (NHS), as well as prevailing philosophies within contemporary society (i.e. the elevation of the individual at the expense of the community/ collective).

Mental health care today

Since the start of the 20th century, the power and status of the medical profession has increased and well over a century later there is now widespread acceptance that they are experts in diagnosing and treating mental health problems. Thus, the medical profession retains its authority over those being treated by mental health services. Psychiatry traditionally subscribes to the bio-medical model; this views mental health problems as pathological and having a biological cause. The model proposes that the cause of mental health problems, and their embodiment in the form of disturbing/distressing thoughts and feelings, resides in the functioning of the brain (i.e. in the form of a chemical imbalance or an inherited disease, etc.). Thus, the bio-medical model sees mental health difficulties as being independent of a person's relationships to the world around them, and to their relationships with others. This model has dominated Western mental health services for well over a century and continues to do so, despite having no supporting systematic body of evidence.

The majority of psychiatrists now recognise that social and psychological factors do play a part in mental health problems. Nonetheless these are often relegated to being of secondary importance to biological factors. The upshot is that the majority of people being treated for mental health problems are given pharmacological treatments, often before being offered any other type of approach. This continues despite the fact that no commonly diagnosed mental health problems (e.g. schizophrenia, bipolar disorder, major depression, anxiety disorders or childhood disorders such as attention deficit disorder) have been proven to be genetic or biological in origin. When we consider that this is the case after many years of intensive research, during which time huge amounts of money, time and energy have been invested, it does beg the question whether there are any to be found. It also makes one wonder whether the bio-medical approach continues to hold such dominance because of the vested interest of the pharmaceutical industry.

Many psychiatrists are also discouraged and disillusioned with the bio-medical model and choose to do further training which employs a psychological approach (i.e. psychodynamic psychotherapy, psychoanalysis, group analysis, systemic therapy, etc.). This searching for an alternative to the bio-medical model can also be witnessed in psychiatric-led groups such as the social psychiatry and anti-psychiatry movements.

We are currently witnessing a sea of change within the NHS and power differentials are shifting in interdisciplinary relationships. Since the 2007 Mental Health Act (MHA) amendments have been implemented, the roles of Approved Clinician (AC) and Responsible Clinician (RC) are no longer restricted to medical practitioners. Instead practitioners from other professions comprising nursing, psychology, occupational therapy and social work may now undertake these roles with overall responsibility for a patient's care. This represents a radical challenge to the view that mental health difficulties are the domain of the medical profession and should be treated accordingly. As Trivedi stated several years ago, 'Perhaps now is the time to really acknowledge the social causes of much mental illness and tackle them, rather than leaving the largely biological discipline of psychiatry to deal with the casualties of social inequalities' (Trivedi 2002, p.82).

Although the majority of mental health services are configured in a way that is biased in favour of formal help, there are alternatives to this model. The following two chapters focus on approaches that harness mutual support. The next chapter considers group approaches to mental health problems including those facilitated by professionals and those that are peer-led. Chapter 6 builds on this by exploring the world of therapeutic communities, organisations that are based on mutual support philosophies where the interface between formal and informal support is clearly acknowledged and employed. It is important to note that despite the strong evidence base supporting therapeutic communities and group approaches they remain in a somewhat marginal position within the mental health field.

CHAPTER 5

Group Therapy

A psychoanalyst named Sigmund Foulkes first introduced group therapy to the UK during the time of the Second World War. Foulkes was also one of the pioneers of the therapeutic community movement (see next chapter). Since then, group therapy has developed and expanded and now includes many different approaches and models that are employed to treat a wide range of mental health difficulties. This chapter will describe some of these approaches and how they are utilised within the field of mental health, as well as the 'curative factors' that have been identified within group therapy.

What is group therapy?

Group therapy involves a group of individuals meeting regularly to share their experiences with the aim of gaining greater insight and understanding, as well as learning new ways to cope with and reduce difficulties. The group is usually facilitated either by one person or more. Depending on the type of group, the facilitator may be professionally trained or not (i.e. in the latter case they may be one of the group members).

This type of therapy builds on the idea that groups are central to human experience and existence. For example, we are born into groups, such as family and culture, and then continue to experience membership of various groups as we proceed through life (e.g. school, activities, work, where we live, etc.). Group therapy harnesses our innate need to be with others who share similar ideas or concerns by providing a place where people are given the opportunity to meet together to share experiences and work through difficulties. This contrasts to individual therapy, which is based on a dyadic relationship with a professional. Despite the extensive practice and literature supporting group therapy, it is commonly regarded as the poor relation to individual therapy. In practice, both types of therapy are equally useful in their respective ways. However, we live in an age that elevates the individual above and beyond the group, and mental health care mirrors this in the way it thinks about and treats mental health problems.

In contrast to individual therapy, groups involve multiple relationships and, therefore, multiple perspectives. They involve both formal *and* informal help, so offer increased therapeutic potential with regard to providing different views and ways of understanding particular experiences. Groups also provide a natural place of learning where there are opportunities for many different types of social interaction, including gaining feedback from others, sharing experiences and coping strategies, reciprocity, social comparison and finding role models (i.e. group members will be at different stages of development and recovery). Receiving feedback from others in the group offers members a unique insight into their own behaviour, including the impact this has on others. Finally, the group provides a safe and supportive forum where new ways of behaving and interacting can be practised, as well as offering a place where group members can form connections with one another and feel a sense of acceptance and belonging. Being with others who are struggling with similar difficulties can help to reduce feelings of isolation and stigma as well as helping to increase self-esteem and confidence. This is especially pertinent to those who are experiencing mental health difficulties.

Curative factors in group therapy

Exploration into curative factors in group therapy has been ongoing for several decades. Yalom (1995) identified 11 'curative factors' or 'primary agents of change' in group therapy:

- *Installation of hope* – Group members are usually at different stages of development/recovery and this provides opportunities for social comparisons. Seeing others improve gives hope that one's own situation can change for the better.

- *Universality* – Realising that others have similar difficulties to oneself can help to normalise and validate these experiences, thus reducing isolation and increasing self-esteem.

- *Imparting information* – Sharing information facilitates understanding of difficulties and can lead to an improvement in coping strategies.

- *Altruism* – This is similar to the idea of the helper-therapy principle in that all group members have opportunities both to receive and offer help. Offering help instils a sense of feeling needed and useful, which can boost self-esteem. This is especially relevant for those experiencing mental health problems where feelings of learnt helplessness and uselessness are commonly held.

- *The corrective recapitulation of the primary family group* – Being a member of a cohesive group can provide greater insight into unhelpful patterns of relating and interacting, as well as guarding against repeating these by learning more helpful and adaptive ways of behaving. For those with attachment difficulties (see Chapter 2) the group is a place where these experiences can start to be challenged and worked through.

- *Development of socialising techniques* – The group provides opportunities to learn and try out new social skills.

- *Imitative behaviour* – This involves learning new and more adaptive ways of behaving through observing others in the group (other group members and the facilitator(s)). This is also known as modelling.

- *Interpersonal learning* – The group provides a forum where members can learn about how they are perceived by others. Yalom talks about the 'adaptive spiral'; this is when what is learnt within the group is transferred to life outside.

- *Group cohesiveness* – The experience of being a group member can provide a sense of belonging and acceptance. In turn this can bring about a reduction in social isolation and alienation. It is proposed that this is the primary therapeutic factor from which all others flow.

- *Catharsis* – Groups provide a space to express and ventilate feelings; this brings relief from emotional distress and can also reduce feelings of guilt and shame.

- *Existential factors* – These include life experiences that are frequently difficult to come to terms with, such as death, isolation and meaninglessness. As trust and openness develops amongst group members these issues can be explored together – this can help to reduce associated anxiety as well as facilitating a greater acceptance of these experiences.

Different types of group

As stated above, group therapy has grown to include many different approaches and models to address a multitude of difficulties, including those relating to both mental and physical health. Despite this diversity, most groups fall into four basic types:

- psychotherapy groups
- activity groups
- psycho-educational groups
- mutual support groups.

These types of group are described in detail below. Pines and Schlapobersky (2000) classified groups by looking at two factors: therapeutic goals (highly specific to non-specific) and group leadership (high level to low level). Figure 5.1 illustrates this by showing examples of how the four different types of groups can be classified according to these criteria:

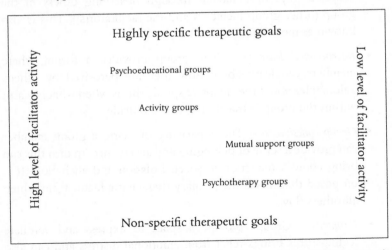

Figure 5.1 A classification of group methods (Pines and Schlapobersky 2000)

Psychotherapy groups

The groups that fall under this heading differ depending on the particular training/school of the facilitator (psychoanalytic, interpersonal, experiential, etc.). However, what psychotherapy groups have in common is the aim of bringing about lasting personality change through non-directive free association. The focus is on self-examination with an exploration of interpersonal interactions and relationships. Psychotherapy groups have a regular meeting time and place; this is generally once a week but can vary. Some groups are time-limited and have a fixed number of sessions, whilst others are ongoing with members joining and leaving from time to time.

Activity groups

These groups help members to focus on particular activities, such as creative pursuits (art, music, writing), cookery, relaxation/meditation, gardening, exercise, movement/dance, and so on. Usually led by professionals such as occupational therapists, art therapists, music therapists or healthcare workers, this type of group can help to foster a sense of connection with others. In addition, these groups can help to build self-confidence and esteem by providing opportunities to achieve something constructive and worthwhile. Activity groups can often be very useful for individuals who find a verbal group too threatening. In this instance, groups that utilise activity can also be used to help prepare the individual for a verbal group by addressing socialisation difficulties and building social confidence. In this way the individual can work on their difficulties and build strengths in a developmental step-wise manner.

Psycho-educational groups

This type of group is usually highly structured with a directive stance being taken by facilitators. For example, the facilitator usually has a didactic role but also gives group members space to think about how this information relates to them and provides opportunities for them to share their experiences with one another. Psycho-educational groups tend to be made up of people who have similar difficulties/experiences and usually work towards clearly defined aims. Some examples include cognitive-behavioural groups for particular difficulties (e.g. depression, anxiety, etc.), voice-hearing groups and anger management groups.

Mutual support groups

Mutual support groups can be traced back to Alcoholics Anonymous and the '12 step programme', founded in the 1930s. It is reported that during the early 1930s an American named 'Roland H' visited the psychoanalyst Carl Jung for help with his alcoholism. Jung concluded he was unable to help him and directed him to the Oxford Group, a religious movement that was popular in the United States and Europe in the early 20th century. Within this group Roland H found others with similar difficulties and through contact with them managed to overcome his alcoholism. He then went on to help others with alcohol problems, and in the late 1930s a breakaway group was formed and named 'Alcoholics Anonymous' (AA). It is estimated that AA now comprises over 100,000 groups.

Mutual support groups are defined as a group of people with similar difficulties who meet regularly to exchange experiences and information and to engage in reciprocal psychological support. These groups are generally based on the valuing of members' experiential knowledge (Borkman 1990). Individuals have often gained valuable knowledge, both from their experience of suffering difficulties and from receiving support. Furthermore, this knowledge can be harnessed and employed for the benefits of the individual and the wider group. An important characteristic of these groups is that they are typically leaderless or run by the group members, and professional involvement is based on a collaborative model. For example, professionals often work with mutual support groups by taking on a supportive role. This may involve a variety of different activities, such as helping with planning and setting up the group, offering support to the facilitators, acting as invited speakers and helping to publicise the group. More detailed information about how professionals can work to benefit mutual support groups is given in Chapter 8.

These groups capitalise on the similarity amongst group members' difficult or stressful experiences to foster the process of mutual support and serve as a temporary personal community that supplements or compensates for difficulties in the participants' natural social networks. As Davison, Pennebaker and Dickerson (2000) state:

...investigations indicate that support groups are particularly valued by individuals whose lives and social identities have been put at risk. A fuller appreciation of the social context of illness enriches our theoretical understandings of social support and social comparison, while offering practical insights about a more appropriate match between health care delivery and the health care sought by patients and their families. (p.216)

A mutual support group is differentiated from a single source of support in that it exposes individual group members to varied ways of reacting and coping with stressful experiences. In addition it is much more difficult to discount or dismiss collective opinion than the views and experiences of an individual. The form these groups may take varies and the increasing numbers of people now using computers has created a burgeoning of Internet-based mutual support groups running alongside more traditional physically based groups.

The functions of mutual support groups are to provide:

- *Social support* – Receiving psychological support from others who understand because they have also experienced similar difficulties leads to a reduction in social isolation and distress.

- *Informational support* – Sharing practical information (i.e. about problems, coping strategies, professional services, available resources, etc.) helps group members to recognise that they have a sense of agency and control over their difficulties.

- *Education* – Through (a) the sharing of experiential knowledge and (b) collaboration with professionals.

- *Advocacy* (optional) – Addressing problems within wider society. For example, many mutual support groups become the springboard for the development of larger-scale movements and foundations.

There are various principles working within mutual support groups. Those set out below are based on *The Self-Help Group Sourcebook* (White and Madara 2002) guidelines:

- *Helper-therapy principle* – Group members have opportunities to both give and receive support. As stated in Chapter 1, Riessman (1965) proposed that having opportunities to help others instils a feeling of self-efficacy and competence. Evidence for this principle has been provided by an observational behavioural measurement of the helping transactions that occur in mutual support groups for people with serious mental health problems, where giving help to others predicted psychosocial adjustment (Roberts *et al.* 1999). In addition, opportunities both to provide and receive support instil a greater sense of wellbeing than being involved in only one of these two processes (Maton 1988).

- *Positive role models* – Group members will be at different stages of recovery. Those who have managed to overcome their difficulties can act as a source of inspiration and support for those who are still struggling.

- *Accessibility* – Mutual support groups are accessible to all, both financially and psychologically. For example, often there is no cost, or a minimal cost to cover expenses. In addition, most groups operate an open format meaning that the group is ongoing and members can choose when they wish to attend. This contrasts with more structured therapy groups where there is often an expectation to attend every meeting.

- *Pooling knowledge/resources* – As group members share their experiences and knowledge, a wealth of important information is pooled which can be subsequently utilised by all individuals attending the group.

- *Acceptance* – Mutual support groups are generally open to everyone and do not have exclusion criteria.

- *Empowerment* – These groups empower their members by giving everybody an equal voice and recognising the unique contribution of each individual. In addition, all group members are given opportunities to be in the position of helper and recipient. This links to the helper-therapy principle described above.

- *Normalisation* – By learning that others have similar difficulties, these experiences are validated and normalised. This can be a powerful corrective experience, especially when the difficulties have been a source of stigma and discrimination.

- *Anonymity* – Participating in a mutual support group does not involve having personal information taken and kept on record.

For many people experiencing mental health difficulties this can be a source of relief and can also result in feeling more able to share information, especially when there is associated shame and embarrassment.

- *Prevention* – George Albee (1982) proposed a 'prevention equation':

$$\text{Incidence of dysfunction} = \frac{\text{Stress} + \text{Constitutional Factors}}{\text{Social Support} + \text{Coping Skills} + \text{Competence}}$$

Mutual support groups reduce the incidence of dysfunction by buffering stress and by enhancing competency to deal with stress. Silverman (1985) points out that stressful life events may not be prevented or avoided, but mutual support groups can act as a powerful modality in the learning of coping skills to deal with these experiences.

- *Options/alternatives generated* – Links to the pooling of knowledge/ resources in that the sharing of experiences can lead to different options and alternatives being generated, which in turn gives the individual choice and empowerment.

- *Turning 'liabilities' into assets* – Mutual support groups can provide a different way of perceiving experiences. In the case of mental health difficulties, the group can transform feelings of discrimination and stigma into acceptance and strength. This transformation occurs through the opportunity to learn a different narrative provided through the collective group experience.

It is clear that mutual support groups can provide an important function within the mental health field where they can be used as an addition to formal support or as a stand-alone intervention, depending on the nature of the difficulties experienced and the individual context. It is important to note that, although mutual support groups cater for a variety of different difficulties, the severity of symptoms and phase of problem development will generally determine whether this type of group is appropriate or not. For example, individuals who are in the initial phase of acute mental health difficulties may be too distressed to be able to benefit from a mutual support group in the first instance. However, once a degree of stabilisation is achieved, mutual support groups can offer much-needed opportunities for socialisation, social support and interpersonal relationships that may not be available elsewhere.

This chapter has outlined the diverse range of therapeutic groups that are available for those wishing to meet others who are experiencing similar difficulties. As detailed, groups help individuals by harnessing the potential power of sharing experiences and supporting one another in this endeavour. The next chapter proceeds to explore a progression of this approach, in the form of therapeutic communities, where group therapy principles are applied to a whole community setting.

CHAPTER 6

Therapeutic Communities

Therapeutic communities can be distinguished from the majority of mental health treatments in that they rely on a combination of both formal and informal help and are built on an understanding of the therapeutic benefits of mutual support. Therapeutic communities involve group therapy but include the additional factor of the community. Whereas the mechanism of change in group therapy is to do with learning new information within the group and applying it to life outside, in therapeutic communities the new information is both learnt and applied within the therapeutic community:

> The basic mechanism of change can be described as this: the therapeutic community provides a wide range of life-like situations in which the difficulties a member has experienced in their relations with others outside are re-experienced and reenacted, with regular opportunities – in groups, community meetings, everyday relationships and, in some communities, individual psychotherapy – to examine and learn from these difficulties. The daily life of the therapeutic community provides opportunities to try out new learning about ways of dealing with difficulties. (Kennard 2004, p.296)

Whiteley and Collis (1987) note that, in some ways, the therapeutic community has similarities with certain methods of family therapy where group meetings at spaced intervals allow the participants to work on the problems outside of the formal group, within the family system. In contrast, these types of interactions outside the formal group would generally be discouraged and regarded as destructive processes in orthodox group psychotherapy. They conclude:

What the therapeutic community has to offer, which circumscribed group therapy does not, is the opportunity to put into practice the insights or realisations gained in therapy and to experiment with new roles and modes of coping in an accepting and understanding social system. It is an ongoing, corrective, emotional experience which, because of its concern with the reality of living together and dealing with real situations as they arise, facilitates a carry-over of personal change from the treatment situation to outside life. (Whiteley and Collis 1987, p.27)

The therapeutic community is described as having an added dimension compared to individual and group therapy (Chazan 2001). Whereas the dyad of individual therapy has a single, linear dimension, and the group is two-dimensional, the therapeutic community is actually three-dimensional in that, despite the fact that the whole community is not present at any point in time, it is constantly present in the therapeutic space. Whiteley (1999) refers to the therapeutic community as a continuous large group.

Therapeutic communities can be traced back to moral treatment, which is described at length in Chapter 4. To recap, moral treatment was founded during the late 18th century at The Retreat in York. Based on the idea that the social environment has a major impact on mental health, moral treatment proposed that people who are experiencing mental health problems require opportunities for social interaction and involvement in meaningful activities. Before moral treatment, people with mental health problems were generally perceived as morally inferior and treated inhumanely. For example, they were often locked up and made to endure physical and mental torture.

Moral treatment also pioneered the idea of rehabilitation. It cannot be overstated how radical an idea this was at the time, owing to the commonly held belief that mental health problems were incurable. Moral treatment countered this and proved to be extremely effective; people started to show improvement rather than remaining the same or getting worse as they had done in the old 'madhouses' and asylums. For a large part of the 19th century, moral treatment was regarded as the gold standard in mental health provision. This changed for a number of different reasons, including the push for building organisations on a much larger scale (thus losing the sense of community so integral to moral treatment), as well as the reluctance of those who founded and developed this approach to take on an expert position. The newly emerging profession of psychiatry had no such qualms and as a result supplanted moral treatment. Another 30 years or so were to elapse before a similar approach to moral treatment emerged in the form of planned environment therapy.

Planned environment therapy

In the 1920s and 1930s, a number of pioneer educationalists began to create liberal therapeutic regimes for disturbed children and adolescents. These ventures, along with many of their successors, are now described under the broad heading of planned environment therapy (PET) (Kennard 2000). The term PET was first employed before the Second World War to describe an approach to living and working with unhappy, deprived, traumatised or delinquent children, young people and adults '...in which all the resources of a thoughtfully created environment, the shared living experience, and above all the enormous healing potential of relationships, are brought together for therapeutic ends' (Planned Environment Therapy Trust n.d.).

The chief initiator behind PET was David Wills, who in 1936 founded and led the Hawkspur Camp, a community for delinquent youths, in collaboration with a child psychoanalyst named Marjorie Franklin. Through her work in various mental hospitals in the 1920s, Franklin became increasingly interested in the relationship between mental health and the environment. Her observations convinced her that when patients were placed in a stimulating environment where support and encouragement were forthcoming, there would be an improvement in their mental health.

Wills was greatly influenced by the work of Homer Lane (1875–1925), an American educator who founded the first community for delinquent adolescents in the UK called the Little Commonwealth. Lane saw emotional disturbance as the product of emotional deprivation. He also believed that the behaviour and character of children improved when they were given more control over their lives. The Little Commonwealth was closed down in 1918 after allegations of misconduct; it has been proposed that a major problem was in Lane trying to fulfil two roles, as head of the community and facilitator of psychoanalytical psychotherapy sessions with the adolescents within the community. Wills was careful not to repeat the same mistake and made sure that he stuck to one role as head of the community, leaving the therapeutic work to others within the organisation.

Wills described the aim of PET as giving children the experience of:

> something on which [they] can absolutely rely, which will never fail, whatever [they] may do. It consists in establishing a relationship such that, however much a child may wound [their] own self-esteem, [they] cannot change the esteem in which we [the staff] hold [them]...when that relationship is established therapy has begun. (Wills 1945, p.65)

Other pioneers working with emotionally disturbed children and adolescents include A.S. Neill, who founded Summerhill School in 1924 (still running today); George Lyward at Finchden Manor; Otto Shaw at Red Hill School; and Melvyn Rose at Peper Harow. These individuals shared a belief that every child or adolescent has a healthy aspect to their personality, but that this may be overtaken by other less healthy aspects such as delinquency or emotional maladjustment through the experience of particular life events. In order for this imbalance to be redressed, they proposed that the child requires nurturing and acceptance within an environment where they can experience emotional support and understanding in order to gain insight into their behaviour and the impact that this has on themselves and others.

PET has many factors in common with adult democratic therapeutic communities. Both hold a belief in the therapeutic benefits of delegating responsibilities, usually taken by professionals/staff, to members of the community in an atmosphere that encourages open expression of feelings and exploration in relationships. In addition, '...both recognise the emotional benefits and opportunity for social maturation which can occur when people have jointly to take responsibility for the community they live in' (Kennard 2000, p.50).

The birth of therapeutic communities

Although moral treatment and PET embody therapeutic community principles, it was not until the time of the Second World War that the term 'therapeutic community' was first used. This is attributed to a psychoanalyst called Tom Main when, in 1946, he described developments at Northfield Military Hospital in Birmingham. During the Second World War, Main, along with a small group of fellow psychoanalysts, including Sigmund Foulkes and Harold Bridger, were involved in what is now known as the 'Second Northfield Experiment'. This built on the work of two other psychoanalysts, Wilfred Bion and John Rickman, who had previously been posted to Northfield. They employed a group dynamic approach in response to the need to rehabilitate traumatised soldiers and return them to duty.

Foulkes and his colleagues were struck by problems of low morale, conflict and disorganisation in the psychiatric wing of the hospital, and had worked hard to overcome this. Main described their approach as:

> an attempt to use the hospital not as an organisation run by doctors in the interests of their own greater technical efficiency, but as a community with the immediate aim of full participation of all its members in its daily life and the eventual aim of resocialization of the neurotic individual for life in ordinary society. (Main 1946, p.67)

A collaborative rather than authoritarian style of staff behaviour was promoted and there was a move away from institutionalising and repressive regimes, towards a more liberal, humane and participative type of culture. Alongside this was the idea of the community as a system needing 'treatment', in contrast to the generally accepted notion that all difficulties are held within the individual.

Parallel to this, a similar development was being pioneered by a psychiatrist called Maxwell Jones at Mill Hill in London (Jones 1968, 1979). Part of London's Maudsley Hospital had been evacuated to Mill Hill at the outbreak of the war, and Jones arrived there in 1940 to head up a small unit in which to study 'effort syndrome'. This was a prevalent condition during wartime in which physical exercise caused people to become breathless and dizzy, and to suffer from palpitations and chest pains. The individuals concerned often convinced themselves that they had a serious heart condition. Jones, a research physiologist by training, set to work to determine the physiological mechanisms underlying the syndrome and decided to introduce a series of lectures aimed at educating the patients about their condition. He reasoned that if they could understand how their symptoms were caused, they might stop worrying that there was something wrong with their hearts.

During this process Jones noticed something remarkable that was to change the course of his life, along with the lives of many others. He began to see a pattern emerge, in that the men who had already completed the course of lectures started to explain what they had learnt to the newly admitted patients, and furthermore became enthusiastic and articulate during this process. Jones recognised that helping one another best helped these individuals, and this had the effect of increasing both their morale and their self-esteem. As a consequence, Jones worked to ensure that there was an atmosphere of open communication, reduced hierarchy and daily structured discussions by the whole unit.

The developments at Northfield and Mill Hill suggested that people experiencing mental health difficulties could be helped more effectively when professionals were willing to be less hierarchical and instead, allowed them to become involved in helping one another. After the war, Main and Jones continued to develop their respective therapeutic community models. In 1946 Main moved from Northfield to become director of the Cassel Hospital in Richmond, Surrey. Meanwhile, Jones was appointed director of a new unit at Belmont Hospital in Surrey. This was later to be renamed the Henderson Hospital and subsequently became the flagship adult democratic therapeutic community. It was also Maxwell Jones whose name became most closely identified with the democratic therapeutic community movement.

The therapeutic community approach

During the 1950s therapeutic community models generated a lot of interest within the mental health field. This was during a time when the old asylum system was still the norm with its straitjackets, padded cells, overcrowding and squalid conditions. Within these asylums, brutality, violence and hopelessness were rife and patients rarely improved. The war was over and there was a need to look towards the future. The National Health Service (NHS) was still in its infancy and a general feeling of optimism pervaded those working within this new organisation. In addition, money was readily available to fund new ideas.

Many of the younger professionals working within mental health were keen to move away from the old repressive and authoritarian regimes. In the therapeutic community model they found evidence that positive change was possible. Medical superintendents such as George McDonald Bell at Dingleton, T.P. Rees at Warlington Park, Duncan Macmillan at Mapperley and David Clark at Fulbourn started to apply therapeutic community principles to their respective hospitals. Clark termed this the 'therapeutic community approach' to distinguish it from specialised units such as the Henderson, the 'therapeutic community proper' (Clark 1965). The latter is now more commonly called the 'democratic therapeutic community'.

The therapeutic community approach was used to great effect with the aim of restoring to patients a more usual pattern of daily living, as well as helping them to develop social relationships with their peers. Some of the common features of these hospitals were group meetings, patient responsibilities and a belief in purposeful activity, as well as the unlocking of wards. This was a far cry from the old regime, and slowly but surely positive change started to occur. The results spoke for themselves, and even the most hardened sceptics became convinced; patients started to improve and emerge as responsible members of the community. Rehabilitation had begun, just as it had all those years ago when moral treatment was introduced.

Therapeutic communities also started to move out of the wards into the community, both in the form of residential and day units. The former included Richmond Fellowship Hostels, Community Housing and Therapy, as well as Threshold in Belfast. The latter included Paddington Day Unit, Marlborough Day Hospital and the Red House in Salford. Another development involved applying these ideas to prisons. HMP Grendon in Buckinghamshire was the first therapeutic community prison to open, in 1962. Based on the Henderson model, it is now part of the controversial 'DSPD' programme – for 'dangerous people with severe personality disorder' (Morris 2004). Over the last 40 years several other prisons have joined HMP Grendon, including a 'fusion' model therapeutic community at Wormwood Scrubs – the Max Glatt Centre. This was run as a democratic therapeutic community but for prisoners with addiction issues (Glatt 1985). In the past, therapeutic communities tend to have been divided into either democratic types (British models) or hierarchical types (American models). The latter are also known as 'concept based', 'behavioural', 'programmatic' and more recently 'addiction' therapeutic communities. These developed in the US in the late 1950s and were set up to help individuals with drug and alcohol addictions. Since then they have spread across the world, and there are now six organisations in various world regions to coordinate activities. There has been ongoing debate as to whether the British and American models may be variations on a common theme with possibilities for theoretical integration, or whether they are actually very different models that share a common name. A concept-based, or addiction therapeutic community, is described as:

A drug-free environment in which people with addictive problems live together in an organized and structured way to promote change toward a drug-free life in the outside community. Every therapeutic community has to strive toward integration into the larger society; it has to offer its residents a sufficiently long stay in treatment; both staff and residents should be open to challenge and to questions; ex-addicts can be of significant importance as role models; staff must respect ethical standards, and therapeutic communities should regularly review their reason for existence. (Broekaert, Kooyman and Ottenberg 1998, p.595)

The above description illustrates the similarities between modern addiction-based models and those of the democratic type. Haigh and Lees (2008) argue that, whereas in the past the differences between the models were more marked, they are now coming together as they face similar challenges connected to the current social and political climate. They discuss how there is a growing emphasis on what the two models can offer one another and give examples of how 'fusion' models are now starting to emerge. In particular, there have been a number of successful fusion therapeutic communities in Europe and Australasia. These illustrate how it is possible to combine strengths from both models as well as offering a promising approach for future development of therapeutic communities.

Alternative asylum and the anti-psychiatry movement

Another group of therapeutic communities grew up around the work of R.D. Laing and David Cooper in the late 1960s and early 1970s. They were both psychiatrists who, through their experiences working within this field, came to oppose the bio-medical model and its associated treatments and founded what is now referred to as the anti-psychiatry movement. The anti-psychiatrists advocated an approach where mental health problems were understood within the psychosocial political context. They argued that the bio-medical model was a means to control individuals who did not fit into the agreed social norms dominant within a particular culture and time, and that psychiatry had manufactured a pseudo-science as a means to gain authority and power. Furthermore, they suggested that society is complicit as it serves to keep those experiencing mental health difficulties separate from the rest of the community.

A number of practical projects grew up out of the anti-psychiatry movement. These shared similarities to the therapeutic community model/approach, but were set up outside the mainstream mental health system as alternative asylums in the true sense of the word. Individuals experiencing mental health problems were offered a place of refuge within a small community, where they were given time and space to explore and work through their difficulties so that healing could ensue. Many of these communities continue through organisations such as the Philadelphia Association and the Arbours Association.

The therapeutic community movement today

Over time, therapeutic communities and therapeutic community approaches have spread, within the UK and overseas, and now cater to a number of different client groups. For example, there are now services for children; children and families; young people and adults. They address a wide range of problems, including severe emotional and social difficulties; complex post-traumatic stress; severe and enduring mental health difficulties; psychosis; eating disorders; addictions and learning difficulties. Provision includes specialist residential units; day services; outreach services; and therapeutic communities set up within the prison system. These exist within both statutory and non-statutory services.

Common attributes of therapeutic communities

The term 'therapeutic community', like 'mutual support', is often used to mean different things, which can be potentially confusing, especially for a newcomer to the area. Despite the diversity found within the therapeutic community field, these services share common principles and aims. They all believe in the importance and therapeutic value of community, and understand mental health difficulties within a social context. In other words, therapeutic communities understand and employ the community as the method or agent of treatment or change.

Haigh *et al.* (2002) define the therapeutic community as:

> a planned environment which exploits the therapeutic value of social and group processes. It promotes equitable and democratic group-living in a varied, permissive but safe environment. Interpersonal and emotional issues are openly discussed and members can form

intimate relationships. Mutual feedback helps members confront their problems and develop an awareness of interpersonal actions. (p.13)

The therapeutic community takes a systems theory stance. Implicit within this is the idea that individual members of the community can be regarded as connected parts of a system, and that all members of the community (staff and clients) have equal responsibilities and status. It also includes the view that mental health difficulties are not located primarily within the individual, but in the network of relationships of which the person is part. Essentially then, the therapeutic community approach is socio-political in that it proposes that personal identity is both dependent upon and in some way constituted by relationships with others. Fundamental to the therapeutic community approach is the process of mutual support. This contrasts to the individualist approach that is currently favoured within mental health treatment.

Community of Communities Quality Network

The Community of Communities Quality Network (C of C) is a standards-based quality-improvement network that was founded by Rex Haigh in 2002. Haigh, a psychiatrist and consultant psychotherapist who has been involved with therapeutic communities for a number of years, wanted to ensure that therapeutic communities were working together to achieve their aims, as well as pooling resources to inform a solid evidence base. The overall aim of C of C is to enable therapeutic communities to evaluate and improve their services by employing methods that reflect their philosophy. To date, two thirds of the UK's therapeutic communities belong to C of C. The network has developed sets of core values and core standards for therapeutic communities, which can be found in Table 6.1 and Table 6.2.

Table 6.1 Core values for therapeutic communities

CV1	Healthy attachment is a developmental requirement for all human beings, and should be seen as a basic human right.
CV2	A safe and supportive environment is required for an individual to develop, to grow or to change.
CV3	People need to feel respected and valued by others to be healthy. Everybody is unique and nobody should be defined or described by their problems alone.
CV4	All behaviour has meaning and represents communication which deserves understanding.
CV5	Personal wellbeing arises from one's ability to develop relationships which recognise mutual need.
CV6	Understanding how you relate to others and how others relate to you leads to better intimate, family, social and working relationships.
CV7	Ability to influence one's environment and relationships is necessary for personal wellbeing. Being involved in decision-making is required for shared participation, responsibility and ownership.
CV8	There is not always a right answer, and it is often useful for individuals, groups and larger organisations to reflect rather than act immediately.
CV9	Positive and negative experiences are necessary for healthy development of individuals, groups and the community.
CV10	Each individual has responsibility to the group, and the group in turn has collective responsibility to all individuals in it.

Table 6.2 Core standards for therapeutic communities

CS1	The community meets regularly.
CS2	The community acknowledges a connection between emotional health and the quality of relationships.
CS3	The community has clear boundaries, limits or rules and mechanisms to hold them in place which are open to review.
CS4	The community enables risks to be taken to encourage positive change.
CS5	Community members create an emotionally safe environment for the work of the community.
CS6	Community members consider and discuss their attitudes and feelings towards each other.
CS7	Power and authority in relationships is used responsibly and is open to question.
CS8	Community members take a variety of roles and levels of responsibility.
CS9	Community members spend formal and informal time together.
CS10	Relationships between staff members and client members are characterised by informality and mutual respect.
CS11	Community members make collective decisions that affect the functioning of the community.
CS12	The community has effective leadership which supports its democratic processes.
CS13	All aspects of life are open to discussion within the community.
CS14	All behaviour and emotional expression is open to discussion within the community.
CS15	Community members share responsibility for one another.

Therapeutic communities in the current climate

The number of therapeutic communities and therapeutic community approaches operating within mainstream mental health services reached a peak in the late 1960s and then started to drop thereafter. By the 1990s they were virtually extinct within the mainstream system due to a combination of changing policies and an emphasis on short-termism within the NHS. As a result, most organisations employing a therapeutic community ethos are now situated within specialist tertiary services or are situated outside the NHS.

One of the biggest challenges for therapeutic communities is the ability to stay alive within the current mental health care climate. In the last 20 years or so there has been a major shift towards parsimony, and the upshot is that all services within mental health are running on extremely tight budgets. Connected to this, services are becoming increasingly short-term. The irony is that in the longer term it is most certainly costing more money, as people are frequently not getting their needs met and subsequently continue to need further treatment, often indefinitely.

Despite this, many therapeutic communities continue to thrive, which is testament to their efficacy in spite of the oppositional climate they face. It is hoped that the C of C will further support and protect these communities. In addition, there are a number of new therapeutic community models emerging, including 'fusion' or hybrid models (i.e. a combination of democratic and addiction models) and those that build on day-treatment models. With regard to the latter, in 2003 the British government published *Personality Disorder: No Longer a Diagnosis of Exclusion* as policy guidance for providers of mental health services to develop suitable treatment for people with personality disorders (NIMHE 2003). The recommendations included the use of therapeutic communities, and as a consequence several non-residential therapeutic communities and services based on the therapeutic community model were set up. Some of these employ innovative techniques using therapeutic community principles, alongside crisis plans and support systems. For example, a number of services operate some face-to-face meetings (from one to five days a week), with member contact outside of these hours via informal meetings, as well as the use of the telephone/internet.

To summarise, the current climate is difficult for therapeutic communities, as these services tend to be more expensive than standard treatments in the short term. However, in the longer term there is growing evidence to demonstrate that therapeutic communities are more cost-effective than standard treatments and a number of cost-offset studies are detailed in the next chapter. Despite this, even the most well-known and respected therapeutic communities face an uncertain future. This can be evidenced by the closure in April 2008 of the Henderson Hospital.

The next chapter explores the evidence base for applied mutual support and focuses on research concerned with therapeutic communities as well as mutual support groups and organisations.

PART III

Applications of Mutual Support

Does Mutual Support Work?

Exploring the Evidence Base

Elsewhere in the book we have learnt about the important role that social relationships play in relation to mental health. Part I detailed how social support correlates with both psychological and physical health, and how our interpersonal relationships impact on the way we view ourselves and relate to others around us. Part II then examined the difference between formal and informal support and looked at how mutual support has been utilised within mental health services. Part III builds on these earlier sections. The next chapter includes detailed information relating to practical applications of mutual support but first there is a need to examine the evidence base further. This chapter focuses on research conducted within two areas that specifically utilise mutual support within their approach; mutual support groups/organisations and therapeutic communities.

In the UK we are becoming increasingly driven by the need to produce evidence to back up intervention choice to ensure that services are both effective and financially viable. In addition, changes within the National Health Service (NHS) mean that services frequently find themselves needing to compete against one another in a bid to secure funding. When we apply this to the two areas we are focusing on in this chapter, both are empirically sound but vary considerably in cost.

In the case of mutual support groups and organisations, these are mainly run on a voluntary basis, so usually do not cost very much to set up and run. However, it is important to remember that these do not take the place of professional services, and individuals accessing mutual support groups and organisations will often require additional professional input. In contrast, therapeutic communities are configured in a way that consists of a combination of peer and professional support within one service. Therapeutic communities are relatively expensive when looked at in the short term, but have proven to be extremely cost-effective when considered from a longer-term perspective. This is detailed later in the chapter. Unfortunately, long-term effectiveness is frequently not taken into consideration due to the emphasis on saving money in the short term. The irony is that pursuing 'cheaper' treatments often results in more money being spent in the long term as people are not receiving appropriate treatment for their needs and so end up requiring more frequent and ongoing input. More importantly, the effect on the individuals concerned can be devastating as they frequently end up feeling increasingly dependent on services as well as more socially isolated within their immediate communities.

Mutual support research

Although interest in mutual support is growing in the UK, the bulk of the research has been conducted within North America where mutual support groups and organisations are well established. One possible reason for this may lie in the difference between our healthcare systems. Unlike the UK, North America does not have an equivalent to the NHS but instead has a combination of privately and publicly funded health care. This results in more limited access to professional healthcare services and so individuals need to be much more proactive in finding alternative ways to address their difficulties. In addition, the recognition of the unique benefits of mutual support groups and organisations increases demand for these interventions.

It is estimated that mental health mutual support initiatives outnumber traditional mental health organisations in the US (Goldstrom *et al.* 2006) and that over 25 million Americans have been involved in mutual support groups at some point in their lives. There is now a substantial literature attesting to the benefits of mutual support, and it has generally been found that more intense and longer-term participation leads to better outcomes. This includes reduced symptoms, reduced use of professional services, shorter hospital admissions, increased coping skills and increased life satisfaction. Additional benefits include better understanding of difficulties leading to increased control, less dependence on services/others and better decision-making with regard to health.

Kyrouz, Humphreys and Loomis (2002) carried out a review of research on the effectiveness of mutual support groups for a number of difficulties, including that of mental health. They focused on groups run by participants who shared similar problems, but also included some studies where the group was co-led by a mutual support peer and a professional or where professionals were involved (either by assisting/advising). The review was concerned primarily with studies that compared mutual support participants with non-participants and/or gathered this information repeatedly over time (i.e. longitudinal studies).

Out of the 45 studies reviewed a diverse range of conditions showed improvements in psychosocial wellbeing, knowledge, mastery, coping and control. For example, Edmunson et al. (1982) followed 80 former mental health inpatients. Half of these individuals participated in a peer-led, professionally supervised mutual support group. At ten months, those who participated in the group had shorter hospital admissions (7 days vs. 25 days) and a higher percentage of group members than non-members were functioning with no contact with the mental health system (53% vs. 23%). Similarly, Galanter (1988) surveyed 356 members of Recovery Inc., a mutual support group for people with mental health difficulties, and found that although approximately half of the sample had been hospitalised before joining, only 8 per cent of group leaders and 7 per cent of recent members had been hospitalised since joining. Kurtz (1988) echoed these findings in her study of the Manic Depressive and Depressive Association. Of the 129 members she interviewed, 82 per cent had been admitted to mental health inpatient services before joining the association, whereas only 33 per cent reported having inpatient admissions after joining. Finally, Roberts et al. (1999) followed 98 individuals who attended GROW group meetings, a self-help organisation for people with long-term mental health problems. Over a period of 6 to 13 months (mean = 8 months) of attendance these individuals showed improved psychological and social adjustments. Adjustment of members who gave and received the most help did not differ significantly from those with lower levels of giving and receiving.

Randomised controlled trials (RCTs) are still considered to be the gold standard in clinical research. The RCT involves randomly allocating people to receive one of several clinical interventions. One of these interventions serves as a control group where either 'treatment as usual' or no treatment is given. Outcomes of other interventions are then compared to the control group. Chien, Thompson and Norman (2008) conducted a RCT which evaluated the effectiveness of a family-led mutual support group in Hong Kong for Chinese caregivers of individuals diagnosed with schizophrenia. The group ran bi-weekly over a period of six months and was compared to standard mental health care treatment. A total of 76 families participated. Results indicated that the mutual support group participants experienced significantly greater improvements in families' burden, functioning and number of support person's, and length of patients' re-hospitalisations. There is increasing evidence that mutual support groups are helpful for caregivers in reducing psychological problems, stress, isolation and guilt, as well as increasing coping mechanisms and interpersonal relationships, both with the care receivers and others (Cook, Heller and Pickett-Schenk 1999; Toseland, Rossiter and Labrecque 1989).

Brown *et al.* (2008) explored how different types of participation in mutual support organisations contribute to recovery. Their findings suggest that involvement in both social roles and leadership roles contribute to recovery, but a socially supportive participation experience maintains a stronger relationship with recovery than an empowering participation experience.

With regard to UK-based research, there have been a number of studies conducted that attest to the benefits of mutual support interventions. Grant *et al.* (2000) conducted a RCT of a formal process that linked GP patients with voluntary mutual support organisations. At four months, 90 referred patients had significantly better scores on seven of nine outcome measures, including anxiety, pain, daily activities and overall health compared with 71 non-referred patients. More recently, Pistrang *et al.* (2008) conducted the first UK review of mutual support groups for mental health. They reviewed 12 empirical studies that explored whether participating in mutual support groups led to improved psychological and social functioning. They concluded that their review provides 'limited but promising evidence that mutual help groups benefit people with three types of problems: chronic mental illness, depression/anxiety, and bereavement' (p.110). Out of the 12 studies, seven reported positive changes for those attending groups. Included within these were two RCTs showing that the outcomes of mutual support groups were equivalent to those of more expensive professional interventions.

Apart from targeting mental health difficulties, mutual support groups are also effective for a wide range of problems that may have associated mental health difficulties. With regard to drug and alcohol problems, research suggests that participating in 12-step or other types of mutual support groups is beneficial in promoting abstinence, which increases with greater group participation (Kelly *et al.* 2006). In the case of terminal illness, Spiegel *et al.* (1989) explored mutual support interventions for women undergoing treatment for metastatic breast cancer. Out of a sample of 86 women, 50 were randomly assigned to have their oncologic care supplemented with a weekly mutual support group. These groups were co-facilitated by a therapist who had breast cancer in remission and a psychiatrist or social worker. On average, support group participants lived twice as long as controls, an average of almost 18 months longer.

It is clear that mutual support groups and organisations are effective in reducing symptoms associated with mental health difficulties. The studies described above illustrate the effectiveness of mutual support groups for both mental and physical health problems, and detail how these interventions can be set up and utilised in different ways. For example, they can be accessed alongside or after receiving professional treatment, or can work as stand-alone services. This will be dependent on the nature and severity of the difficulties experienced, as well as the phase of symptom development (i.e. acute onset, chronic, remission, etc.).

Therapeutic communities research

People who seek treatment within therapeutic communities have usually had contact with other services. In many cases therapeutic community treatment is sought as a last resort when other interventions have tried and failed. There are a number of possible reasons for this including the fact that therapeutic communities are often misunderstood or not considered due to the approach being significantly different to that employed within mainstream mental healthcare services. Linked to this, there is also the issue of cost and funding. Due to the purchaser/provider split within the NHS and frequent overspending, it is usual for the least expensive services to be sought out. These calculations are commonly made with regard to the short term, and unfortunately it is rare for longer-term outcomes or cost to be taken into consideration.

Outcome studies

The early research on therapeutic communities was descriptive, mostly comprising single-case studies, and conducted by therapeutic community practitioners (Bion 1960; Foulkes 1948; Jones 1968; Main 1946). Gradually, more sociological, anthropological studies began to be carried out, usually by people outside of the therapeutic community field (Rapoport 1960).

As funding for services has become increasingly linked to outcomes, the attempt to explore the effectiveness of therapeutic communities has become an urgent issue. In 1998, a systematic international review of therapeutic community effectiveness was commissioned by the High Security Psychiatric Services Commissioning Board. This focused primarily on in-treatment and post-treatment outcome for people with a diagnosis of personality disorder in democratic therapeutic communities. It also included relevant in-treatment and post-treatment outcome studies of the effectiveness of concept-based therapeutic communities, usually for substance abusers and particularly those in secure settings (Lees, Manning and Rawlings 1999). The review collated a substantial enough number of good quality studies to allow a meta analysis to be conducted (Lees, Manning and Rawlings 2004). This analysis, taking careful account of sources of heterogeneity and possible publication bias, showed a clear and positive treatment effect for therapeutic communities. According to the UK National Service Framework for Mental Health, this study fits the criteria for Type I evidence (i.e. at least one good systematic review, including at least one RCT).

Although there is a growing body of research exploring the effectiveness of therapeutic communities, the question of how therapeutic communities work is still largely unanswered. Lees *et al.* (2004) see this as being due to difficulties in teasing out the different mechanisms at work inside such a complex and multi-faceted treatment.

Curative factors in therapeutic communities

Compared with the curative factors in group therapy, the curative factors in therapeutic communities have received less attention. In order to address this, Whiteley and Collis (1987) conducted a study with patients at the Henderson Hospital. They found that learning from interpersonal actions, acceptance (especially in the early stages of treatment) and self-understanding were the most prominent therapeutic factors as categorised from patients' accounts of the 'most important event' in the previous week. It is interesting to note that in this study, half of the most important events reported by patients took place outside the setting of formal therapy groups but largely within the boundaries and life of the community. This again illustrates the importance of informal helping and support.

Mutual support within the therapeutic community

The therapeutic community literature makes many references to mutual support. This is not surprising considering the central position that this type of support has within therapeutic communities. As one of the founders of the therapeutic community movement wrote, '...the most important lesson that therapeutic communities have shown [is] the importance of the "patient's" own peer group' (Jones 1979, p.6). Despite this, there has been a lack of systematic research directly examining mutual support processes in therapeutic communities. This is probably due to the fact that mutual support is such an integral part of therapeutic community treatment that it has not been investigated as a separate factor worthy of exploration in its own right.

There have been a number of anecdotal accounts, both from people who have been resident in therapeutic communities and those who have worked as staff within these organisations that allude to the importance of mutual support. Drahorad (1999) reported on experiences of ex-patients of the Cassel Hospital, one of whom, Sue, says:

> ...what was most significant to me was that whatever I was beginning to feel, the routines, the structures but most importantly the people, patients and staff alike, were still around me. However awful and pathetic I felt within myself I still had a place which I belonged to and where I felt recognised and accepted. This realisation came to me as a huge relief. (p.203)

Similarly, an ex-member of the Arbours, a therapeutic community founded in 1970, reflected on her experience as '...what has worked for me in Arbours is living with other people and struggling with the difficulties I've had with them, and them with me' ('Matilda', quoted in Berke, Masoliver and Ryan 1995, p.21).

There have also been case studies such as that conducted at the Cassel Hospital exploring patients' perceived experience of life in the Family Unit (Biggs 1987). Thirteen inpatients and 17 ex-patients were interviewed from a total of 25 families. The findings highlight the fundamental importance of mutual support to these individuals.

For example, participants reported feeling a sense of relief and safety in being welcomed by other patients who were expected to support them. In addition, for many participants it was a significant discovery to find that they could help and support others. Interestingly, those participants who were inpatients at the time of being interviewed were very concerned about their relationship with staff, whereas ex-patients spoke more about their interaction with other patients. The longer they had been away, the more they spoke of the mutual support they had experienced. In addition, they reported that their confidence was more often increased by contact with other patients than with staff.

A handful of studies have explored the impact of therapeutic community treatments on substance abusers' social support networks. According to the therapeutic community approach, social affiliation with the drug-free peer community is the basis for patients initiating therapeutic change (De Leon 2000). The findings of two studies lend support to this idea. Dermatis *et al.* (2001) conducted a study with 322 residents in a therapeutic community for substance abusers. After controlling for socio-demographic characteristics, perceived benefit of therapeutic community treatment was associated with greater therapeutic community member affiliation, whereas level of depression was inversely correlated with this. More recently, another study found that individuals who completed therapeutic community treatment had larger social support networks and more close friends, reported greater satisfaction with the support they received, and were more willing to utilise support resources (Richardson 2002).

These allusions to mutual support within therapeutic communities led me to conduct a qualitative study to explore these processes further (Loat 2006). This research was conducted at the Cassel where I interviewed 12 individuals about their experiences of mutual support whilst they were resident there. I analysed the interviews using interpretative phenomenological analysis (IPA: Smith and Osborn 2003), a structured method for systematic and detailed analysis of qualitative data. IPA was specifically designed to enable the exploration of participants' experiences from their own perspective rather than from that of the researcher (Willig 2001). Eight themes, each comprising a number of sub-themes, were identified from the analysis and these were organised into three higher-order domains. These related to participants' experiences of being in the therapeutic community; the process of giving and receiving mutual support; and the impact of mutual support on their sense of self and perception of their difficulties. These are listed in Table 7.1. Overall, participants' experiences of mutual support were positive, and the study identified a number of ways in which these processes operated within the therapeutic community and the impact these had on individual members. The findings are consistent with the mutual support literature, providing further evidence for the benefits of this type of support. The outcome of the study highlights the importance of providing people experiencing mental health difficulties with opportunities to support one another, alongside the provision of professional support.

Table 7.1 Research findings from exploration of mutual support processes in a therapeutic community (Loat 2006)

Domains	Themes	Sub-themes
Context	(1) Journey into the unknown	Shock and surprise Feelings of uncertainty
	(2) A different approach	How will it work? Usefulness of therapeutic community approach
Processes of support	(3) Struggling together	'Nice to know you're not the only one.' 'It makes you listen.' Feeling understood Reciprocity
	(4) What I do affects others	Others are suffering too Looking in a mirror
	(5) Others care about me	'Not being alone' 'Patients care because they want to'
	(6) Being accepted	'You're not judged' 'People like me for who I am'
Impact of Support	(7) 'Making me feel human again'	'I am worth something' 'Helping others helps me'
	(8) There is hope	'If they can do it...I can do it too'

Finally, it is important to include some research findings exploring the cost-effectiveness of therapeutic communities. Dolan *et al.* (1996) compared service usage (mental healthcare inpatient, day patient, outpatient and periods of imprisonment) of 24 patients at the Henderson Hospital for one year pre- and post-treatment. In the one year before admission these patients had each used an average of £13,966 worth of mental healthcare and prison services. In the one year following discharge, the same patients each used an average of only £1308 of services. Thus, pre-admission costs had been reduced by nine-tenths. This represents a cost-offset of £12,658 per patient. Thus, the average £25,000 cost of treatment at the Henderson would be recouped within two years and represent a saving thereafter.

Davies, Campling and Ryan (1999) reported similar findings when they compared 52 individuals diagnosed with severe personality disorder treated at Francis Dixon Lodge in Leicester, three years pre- and post-treatment. Following treatment psychiatric bed use dropped from 74 days per year to 7.2 for the patients referred from outside the district, and from 36 days per year to 12.1 for those locally based. This represents an average cost-offset of £8571 in the first year following treatment for those patients referred from outside the district. By comparing referrals from within and outside their own area, they also suggested that a local service may have a preventive cost-offset function. For example, referring individuals at an earlier point prevents further inappropriate use of other resources. Haigh (2002) states:

> An extension of the cost-offset argument would be to claim that a number of these patients do not need residential treatment, and there would be clinical and social advantages to treating them without removing them from their normal environment – in locally accessible day units. The costs of treatment in such units would be significantly less, and rehabilitation could be designed as an integrated part of the programme. The development and use of such modified therapeutic communities, including outreach elements and treatment in day units, has been proposed. (p.66)

In summary, it is clear that there is strong evidence to support the efficacy and effectiveness of both therapeutic communities and mutual support groups and organisations for the treatment of mental health difficulties. Despite this, they remain in a somewhat marginalised position within the mental health field. Finding services that employ mutual support is currently not a simple or straightforward task, within the UK at least. The next chapter attempts to address this and provides a guide to those seeking mutual support and for those who are interested in providing and facilitating such interventions.

CHAPTER 8

Putting Theory into Practice
How to Make a Difference

This chapter is divided into two main sections. The first, 'Accessing mutual support', provides information for those experiencing mental health difficulties to help them decide whether mutual support is the most appropriate and useful way forward. It outlines different issues for potential mutual support group members to be aware of and finishes with recommendations as to how to identify and access reputable groups.

The second section, 'Providing mutual support', is aimed at those interested in facilitating mutual support interventions. It includes advice on the setting up and delivery of mutual support groups as well as ways to incorporate mutual support principles into clinical practice.

Mutual support groups are led and facilitated by non-professionals, but frequently involve collaboration with professionals. A well set-up group will be mindful of the need for members to own the group and to make decisions together but will also draw on the support of professionals when needed (e.g. to help with the initial setting up of the group and then provide ongoing advice and assistance as and when necessary). This chapter is written with this joint-working model in mind.

Accessing mutual support

Why mutual support?

First, it is important to clarify why you are interested in accessing mutual support and what you are hoping to gain from it. The following questions can act as a useful guide – you may wish to keep a record of your responses, as they can be helpful to refer back to at a later stage:

- What is it about mutual support that interests you? Try to identify as many different ideas as you can.

- What are you hoping to gain from a mutual support group?

- Why mutual support rather than another type of support/ intervention?

- How does mutual support differ from other types of support/ interventions you have tried?

- Have you got the necessary time and energy to commit to attending a mutual support group?

- Do you wish to share your experiences with peers and hear about their experiences?

- Do you have any other support from elsewhere?

Being clear about what you are looking for can help to decide whether a mutual support approach is going to be useful. It can also be useful to discuss this with others if possible. There is little research exploring who is most likely to benefit from mutual support interventions, so the information detailed below is important to think about when considering whether mutual support is the most appropriate intervention for you at this stage.

Importance of professional involvement

If your difficulties are affecting you to the extent that you are unable to proceed with your regular day-to-day life, I strongly recommend that you first make an appointment with your General Practitioner (GP). It may be that you need to speak to a mental health professional – your GP can advise about this. I am recommending this as a necessary first step to ensure that you receive appropriate treatment for the difficulties you are experiencing. It is also important that any potential underlying physical problems are explored and ruled out. Following this consultation, and the subsequent outcome, you may then wish to proceed with finding a mutual support group/service. Again, this can be discussed further with professionals who should be able to advise.

Severity of difficulties

Generally the more severe the difficulties, the more important it is that professional help is first sought out. When problems are in an acute phase it can sometimes be difficult to make use of a group and it may be more helpful to wait until you feel stable enough to be able to utilise and benefit from a mutual support approach.

Pros and cons of mutual support

There are pros and cons to all interventions and it is no different with mutual support. Below are some of the potential benefits as well as some of the possible dangers of mutual support. Being aware of the latter in advance can help to reduce the likelihood of these occurring.

Potential benefits of mutual support:

- meeting others with similar experiences
- sharing experiences and understanding
- reduction in social and emotional isolation
- realising that you are not alone
- sense of belonging
- social interaction/support
- learning from others in a similar position
- sharing coping strategies
- offering support – promotes feelings of self-efficacy/confidence
- opportunities for social comparisons – instillation of hope and inspiration.

Possible dangers of mutual support:

- receiving inappropriate advice from others
- negative social interactions
- anti-professional attitudes
- taking on too much
- helping others as a way of avoiding own issues
- experience of seeing others struggling

- worrying about other group members
- difficulties accepting support of peers
- experience of others refusing your help
- forming close attachments and having to deal with endings (i.e. others/oneself leaving group).

Finding reputable mutual support groups/organisations

After considering and working through the above, if you feel ready to attend a mutual support group, it is important to ensure it is reputable as well as being run in a safe and supportive manner. In the appendices of this book there are details of organisations both within and outside the UK that may be of help. It is also worth seeking out local knowledge and contacting specialist organisations that deal with the types of difficulties that you are experiencing:

- *Local knowledge* – Ask around. For example, local services such as GP surgeries, health clinics, community centres, etc. often have information about local groups and organisations. If this information is not forthcoming, make an appointment with your GP to discuss this with them directly. Even if they do not have this information to hand, they should be able to look into this for you. If you manage to obtain details about a local group, get in touch with the contact person to find out more information.

- *Specialist organisations* – It is worthwhile exploring whether there are specialist organisations/societies that are set up to deal with the particular problems you are experiencing. If so, they often have knowledge about groups and meetings in your local area. Failing this, they may be able to put you in touch with other people experiencing similar difficulties.

Once you find a group it is important to try and commit to it for a decent period of time in order to evaluate whether it is going to be helpful or not. At first it will probably feel new and slightly strange, especially if you are not used to a group approach. Like any intervention, change will probably not happen immediately and will require time and effort. However, as stated, the evidence suggests that this will be rewarded in that mutual support groups have been shown to offer positive outcomes for those who are willing to invest in them.

Providing mutual support

This section is aimed at those of you who are interested in setting up and delivering mutual support groups. It also provides information as to how principles of mutual support may be employed in general clinical practice.

Setting up a mutual support group

AIMS OF THE GROUP

Being clear about the aims of the group is important with regard to planning, enlisting the support of others and advertising to potential members. It helps if the aims are simple and concise rather than over-inclusive and wordy. Some examples are:

'The _____ group aims to provide individuals who experience _____ opportunities to meet others in a similar situation and provide mutual support.'

'To enable people experiencing _____ to meet others in a similar situation on a regular basis to provide mutual support.'

'YOU ALONE CAN DO IT BUT YOU CANNOT DO IT ALONE...'

Fitting with the philosophy of mutual support, do not try to do everything yourself! After clarifying the aims of the group, the next step is to find out if there are other people who may be interested in collaborating. For example, are there professionals (i.e. psychologists, medics, nurses, occupational therapists, etc.) who may be able to help? In addition, are there other groups/organisations that may be able to offer help in areas such as providing advice and support, identifying appropriate professionals and advertising the group?

PLANNING MEETINGS

Once interested individuals have been identified, it is important that you arrange a series of regular meetings to discuss and decide what needs doing in order to get a group up and running. This initial planning phase is a vital period with regard to ensuring that the group is set up properly and stands the best chance of success, so make sure that you allow enough time for this to happen. During these meetings you will need to agree on roles and responsibilities for those involved. These may include positions such as chair, secretary, liaison officer, public relations/ publicity officer, etc., and the forming of a committee/working party. Meetings need to be structured to include introductions (for any new members), agenda, minutes from previous meeting, including feeding back on action points that were agreed and identifying new action points that need to be taken forward. With regard to the latter it is vital that these are well defined and that it is clear who is taking responsibility for what.

FINDING A SUITABLE GROUP VENUE

When looking for an appropriate venue the following need to be considered:

- *Location* – Is it easy to get to? Is it situated near to public transport? Is there anywhere to park?

- *Accessibility* – Is the location/venue fully accessible for all? For example, is it suitable for those who require wheelchair access?

- *Practicalities* – Is the room a suitable size for the numbers you are planning to accommodate? Is it quiet/private/comfortable? Are there enough chairs? Is there access to public conveniences/ kitchen?

- *Cost* – If there is a charge, find out exactly how much this will be and then a decision needs to be made with regard to how this will be met. Often the fairest way is to share the cost amongst the group. If this is not possible, funding needs to be sourced from elsewhere.

ADVERTISING/PUBLICITY

Advertising and publicity are vital in ensuring there are enough individuals who know about and wish to attend the group. There are a number of ways that this can be done, including contacting local newspapers/ radio/television stations; national/local societies and organisations; National Health Service (NHS) (GP surgeries, health centres); non-statutory services and service-user groups/forums. In addition, posters can be put up in many of the above services or venues, as well as around the local area (community centres, libraries, supermarkets, pharmacies, local notice boards, etc.). Word of mouth is also an important, and often overlooked, method of advertising. Any publicity needs to include:

- information about the group (i.e. aims and objectives)
- date, time and venue of first meeting
- name and telephone number of contact person.

Facilitating a mutual support group

Some groups have a designated facilitator/facilitators, whilst other groups rotate this position. In the case of the latter, this is usually only introduced once the group is established. For example, when a group is in its infancy it is vital that there are named facilitator(s) to undertake this role in order for the group to feel safe and contained, otherwise there is increased likelihood that people will leave and the group will fragment.

CREATING A SAFE AND SUPPORTIVE GROUP

When people start to attend a group they usually have a variety of hopes, fears and uncertainties. An important part of the group facilitator role is to create a safe and supportive space for group members to enable the development of trust and membership in the group. The role of the facilitator can be demanding and challenging at times, and it is vital that appropriate support and supervision is in place for whoever undertakes this position.

The facilitator needs to be clear about where and when the group takes place to help create a sense of structure and containment. It is important to have regular meetings, and it is usually helpful to have these on the same day and at the same time. During the first session the group needs to agree on how often they wish to meet as well as dates and times for future meetings. It is useful to review the frequency of the meetings on a regular basis, as it is sometimes difficult to gauge the most appropriate intervals during a first meeting. In addition, consideration needs to be paid to the fact that groups, and group needs, change over time and what suits the group at one point in time may not be the case at a later stage.

Prior to each meeting the facilitator(s) need(s) to prepare the room, as the way that the room is organised is important with regard to how the group functions. For example, having chairs arranged in a circle helps to enable clear verbal and non-verbal communication and also creates a sense of democracy. It is also important that the room is comfortable (i.e. temperature, light, noise, etc.). Connected to this, a decision needs to be made as to whether refreshments are provided or not during the meeting. Some groups provide drinks/biscuits during the meeting and other groups tend to provide these during a break or at the end. Again, it is best if the group makes these decisions in order to promote collaboration and a sense of group ownership.

Confidentiality needs to be acknowledged and implemented. It is vital that group members feel able to share information and know that it will stay within the group as this helps to build trust; in turn this helps to create a cohesive group. However, it is also important to discuss when confidentiality may need to be waived; for example if there are issues around risk.

At the beginning of each group meeting the facilitator(s) should begin with introductions. This ensures that everybody knows each other and helps to develop connections between group members. Sometimes name badges are worn to help in this respect.

Facilitators need to give information about the aims of the group and what it can offer. This should be done in collaboration with group members. In addition, it is important for group facilitators to be clear about the limitations of the group. For example, the group can provide mutual support but cannot replace mental health and medical care. There may be times when support needs to be sought from outside the group, and this is the individual's responsibility.

It is also important to find out what group members want from the group, in order to ensure that the group is meeting the needs of its members. Also it is useful to work in collaboration with the group members when setting group rules and boundaries in order to increase empowerment and group ownership. Some examples of group rules, sometimes known as 'ground rules' or 'ways to help the group feel safe', are:

- start and finish on time

- introductions at the beginning

- one person speaking at a time

- respect for other people's views

- confidentiality

- no physical/verbal aggression.

Facilitators also need to be mindful of modelling appropriate behaviour to group members. Some examples include open and clear communication, listening to others, being respectful and sensitive, good time-keeping, etc.

STRUCTURING THE GROUP

The type of group will determine to what extent the group needs to be structured. It is generally accepted that more structure and focus is required for people whose experiences are more fragmented. It may be useful to set a specific amount of time for specific tasks within each meeting, and this needs to be agreed by the group. Examples of structuring include:

- introductions at beginning
- greetings and welcoming new members
- stating purpose of group
- reviewing ground rules
- sharing information that may interest group (i.e. events, talks, etc.)
- discussion
- summing up and ending
- reminder about date and time for next meeting.

At the first meeting, group members and facilitators need to agree the purpose of the group – why are we here and what do we wish to achieve? Is the group's aim to provide mutual support exclusively or also to provide information? Does the group need the collaboration of professionals? Do invited speakers need to be brought in? Other questions that need to be decided at the first meeting include:

- What is the name of the group?
- Is the group going to be open or closed?
- How long should meetings be?
- When and how often should meetings take place (time/day/ dates)?

There is also a need to ensure that there is a designated person who has contact details of all group members in case of any difficulties (e.g. if meeting needs to be cancelled, etc.). Finally, group members should agree on when the group will be reviewed.

Choosing topics for meetings is something that can be used to help keep the group focused and to ensure that meetings are used effectively. Again, it is important that the group works together to decide on these. One possible way of doing this is to ask the group to spend some time thinking together and to make a list of possible topics. A vote can then be taken on which ones the group feels would be most useful.

EVALUATING/REVIEWING

It is vital that the group is reviewed regularly in order to ensure that it is working as well as it can. The best way of doing this is through the employment of questionnaires, as these can be kept anonymous in order to ensure that group members feel free to answer honestly. When putting questionnaires together it is important to ensure that questions are phrased in a way that invites an open-ended response, rather than being closed (i.e. yes/no responses) as this will provide more detailed and useful information. Possible areas that you may wish to cover could include:

- checking whether venue/day/time/frequency are OK
- whether group members feel welcome
- whether they find the group helpful
- what they feel works well
- what they think needs to be improved
- what topics they would like to see addressed in the future
- whether they feel they have opportunities to say what they wish in meetings
- feedback about group size.

Those running the group then need to go through all questionnaires and collate this information. A meeting should then be arranged for this information to be fed back and discussed within the group; this can then be used to discuss whether any changes need to be made. If the group is not agreed on these then a vote can be taken.

Professional input

As previously stated, the model I recommend is one where the group is led and facilitated by non-professionals, but has the support and input from professionals as and when required. There are a number of different ways that professionals can be involved in mutual support and some ideas are presented here.

IDENTIFYING LOCAL GROUPS AND MAKING CONTACT

Be aware of local mutual support groups and ensure that you make contact with them. For example, exchange contact details, request copies of their literature, subscribe to newsletters and ensure they are disseminated within your service. Making this contact can be of mutual benefit; individuals who use your service may start to attend the group and the group may require professional input from you.

OFFERING TO PROVIDE INPUT

Offer to provide speaking engagements and/or training to local groups. The former can help to ensure that groups are provided with professional knowledge and expertise about particular issues/difficulties. In addition, training and supervision can be provided to group facilitators and those involved in running the group. For example, this could be connected to setting up and running groups, or how to manage specific difficulties.

NETWORKING/COLLABORATION

It is important to develop networking with regard to meeting group needs for speakers, advisors, referrals, researchers, training, consultants, etc. Working collaboratively with groups can be mutually beneficial and involves reciprocity. As well as professionals offering their support to groups, ensure that groups are invited to your service to present what they are doing to staff and service users.

EDUCATING AND ADVOCATING

Educate other professionals about the value of mutual support groups and share information about what is available in the local community. In addition, it is important to advocate for increased awareness and understanding of mutual support groups. This could include giving presentations to colleagues/other services; compiling a directory of local and national groups, etc. Identify the need for new groups in your local area and educate others with regard to developing a potential group.

INCORPORATING MUTUAL SUPPORT IDEAS INTO GENERAL CLINICAL PRACTICE

In addition to the above ways of getting directly and indirectly involved in mutual support groups, it is also important to think about how you might try to incorporate mutual support principles and ideas into your own clinical practice. This can be achieved in a number of different ways but starts with recognition of the immense wealth of information and expertise that service users hold. Weaving this into your practice by helping service users also to become aware of this can be extremely beneficial. You may wish to develop structured ways in which these principles can be applied, such as setting up opportunities for service users to share experiences and to provide support to one another. This can be done through incorporating space to do this within existing groups, such as through community meetings or service user forums, or through the development of a mutual support group within the service.

I hope that the information within this chapter has provided some stimulation to facilitate the application of mutual support ideas. It is important to remember the principle behind mutual support when trying to put some of these ideas into practice, that 'you alone can do it but you cannot do it alone'…in other words, seek out the support of others rather than trying to do everything by yourself.

The next, and final, chapter builds on what we have previously discussed to explore the future of mutual support.

CHAPTER 9

The Future of Mutual Support

In the previous chapters we have learnt about the important role that mutual support plays in mental health. Despite the evidence attesting to this, the majority of mental services continue to treat mental health difficulties from an individual perspective, paying little attention to mutual support or to the social context.

This is particularly relevant when we look at the current crisis in mental health provision. As we proceed into the 21st century, mental health problems continue to grow whilst services struggle to keep up with demand. The National Health Service (NHS) is currently stretched to capacity and ongoing funding cuts make this situation increasingly difficult to manage. As a result, services have been reconfigured to provide shorter-term services, but the upshot is that people frequently end up relapsing and requiring longer-term support due to their difficulties being inadequately addressed. The dominant perspective within the Western world views mental health as an individual phenomenon, and services therefore tend to approach and treat mental health difficulties as such. Consequently, there is frequently very little thought given to the impact and importance of the social context and to social support, which is so vital to mental health.

This lack of adequate treatment and disregard of the social context creates a situation where individuals become (a) dependent on services (as they are not making full recoveries) and (b) socially isolated. The combination of these two factors results in many individuals who experience mental health problems becoming segregated from wider society and ending up in the role of 'professional patient'. When Care in the Community was first introduced in the early 1990s it employed a rhetoric that suggested it was about integrating those experiencing mental health difficulties back into communities outside of mental health service settings. In reality it has involved moving people out of hospital settings into pseudo communities where mental health difficulties are frequently viewed with a mixture of anxiety and fear.

A key issue that Care in the Community has failed to consider is the discrimination and stigma attached to mental health and how this keeps those labelled with such difficulties from fully integrating into the world outside of mental health services. In addition, services compound this due to the emphasis being placed on maintenance and improvement rather than recovery. This links to the points made earlier concerned with the short-term nature of service involvement. Services operate according to short-term plans, with the result that individuals tend to be shunted from one short-term service to another. This presents a fundamental challenge to the recovery process in that it prevents service users from forming any lasting connections and relationships with others necessary for any meaningful social integration to occur. When we consider the social alienation and isolation frequently experienced by those suffering mental health difficulties, it becomes clear that mental health services need to widen their scope to include the social context if they are serious about addressing these problems.

Over the course of the previous chapters we have explored the fundamental reasons why the social context is so important to mental health. In Chapter 2 we looked at how attachment affects mental health, and in particular how attachment difficulties in childhood are correlated with a wide range of mental health problems. In Chapter 3 we then explored how mental health difficulties can negatively affect social relationships and how many people with these experiences can end up in socially-isolated positions. When we apply this to mental health provision it is clear that the current configuration of service delivery is going to exacerbate these problems further. This is because we are essentially expecting people to keep moving from one service to another, usually at the point when they are starting to improve and to feel comfortable with the people around them. This process is meant to prevent dependency and promote person-centred recovery, in that improvement equals time to 'move on'. However, in reality, the process frequently results in the opposite – that is, it compounds dependency and prevents recovery as it essentially re-traumatises those who are trying to work through attachment difficulties by moving them to a new service before they are ready and able to make this transition. The result is that many individuals end up imprisoned within socially-isolated positions as a way of protecting themselves from this process. In fact, what we now have is a parallel 'community' of mental health service users who in the main are separated from the rest of the population with little thought given to their social context and to the quality of their relationships with others.

Alongside this, there are issues around power and disempowerment that need to be considered. We discussed this in Chapter 4 when we explored the power differential within mental health services and how in many ways mental health provision can be driven by defensive practice and a need to assert control over the behaviour of others. We learnt about how this power differential increases with the service's perception of the seriousness of the problem. One example is the legal detention of individuals in hospital and how they are required to stay connected with community mental health services when they leave so that their medication and functioning can be monitored. With the introduction of Community Treatment Orders (CTOs) under the Mental Health Act 2007, this has become a much more contentious issue, as individuals who have been detained in hospital under the Act can be discharged under a CTO and be immediately recalled to hospital should they decide to disagree with their treatment plan. When these factors are considered within the context of the social marginalisation that many people diagnosed with mental health difficulties encounter, it is not difficult to understand the disenfranchised position that these individuals frequently end up in.

From the perspective of someone who has worked as a mental health professional in both inpatient and community settings, it is clear that the current approach to mental health is not working to the advantage of those it is designed to be helping, and that an important factor in the recovery process is missing. In the preceding chapters we have learnt about the importance of social and mutual support, to both mental and physical health. Despite the overwhelming evidence attesting to the vital function these supportive interactions provide, they remain an overlooked and undervalued factor within mental health services.

Yet this was not always so; looking back over the history of mental health care we discovered how mutual support was once central to mental health provision in the form of 'moral treatment'. We also learnt how moral treatment proceeded to be displaced by the newly formed psychiatric profession, which introduced a very different way of understanding and treating mental health difficulties. Whereas moral treatment was concerned with collaboration and mutual support, the medical profession was intent on taking an authoritarian, custodial stance. As a result, they wasted no time in introducing a taxonomic system whereby mental health difficulties were categorised at an individual level and treated using a combination of physical and chemical means. Clearly this approach gives little thought to the individual's social context and, if considered, it is usually subsequent and secondary to a medication regime. The latter is often given with the clear message that this needs to be an ongoing treatment. This propagates the idea that mental health difficulties are 'for life', and the result is that people remain locked into this mentality and the associated expectations of what this means.

If the pioneers of moral treatment had taken up the position of 'expert' rather than letting the fledgling psychiatrists take on this role, then history might have taken a very different turn. Equally, if moral treatment had continued to be the dominant model, then mental health provision, and indeed the world around it, would be a very different place. I say this because if the principles underpinning moral treatment formed the basis of how we understand and approach mental health difficulties, then the socially constructed divide that separates those experiencing mental health difficulties from those who are not would have no reason to exist, and the associated stigma, discrimination and disempowerment would fall away with it. When we stop to reflect on this divide, it is clear that one of its functions is as a defence against the reality that we are all vulnerable to mental health problems. By creating a segregated group who we class as 'mentally ill', we can pretend that these individuals are different to us, that they require special treatment and need to be separated from the rest of society. This construct keeps people who experience mental health problems in a position where they end up seeing themselves in this way. For example, people who experience long-term mental health problems are frequently regarded as being incapable of working and being unable to provide anything of value to the community, with the result that they accept this view as being true. In other words, certain learnt behaviours and self-fulfilling prophecies are created and maintained where the individual believes that they have nothing valuable to offer. This has a significant negative impact on self-esteem and the ability to move towards wellness and recovery.

In Chapter 2 we learnt about how our sense of self is constructed by our relationships and interactions with those around us. The way in which mental health difficulties are perceived is also influenced by the social context, and this can be illustrated by exploring how similar experiences have been understood in different ways by different cultures at different points in history. For example, in the Middle Ages mental health difficulties were termed 'madness' and perceived as a moral issue, such as a punishment for sinning or as a test of faith. Similarly, during the late 19th century and throughout most of the 20th century it was standard for homosexuality to be viewed pathologically. In fact, it was only declassified by the American Psychiatric Association as a 'mental disorder' in 1973, and it has now been decriminalised in nearly all developed countries.

The French philosopher Michel Foucault proposed that, within the Western world, discourses of mental health have changed significantly over the past two centuries. He links this to the changing power relationships and interests of particular groups and points out that unchanging 'facts' do not exist; instead the reality is that there are changing social constructions. Clearly, these affect the way that we perceive and understand different phenomena, including those relating to experiences and behaviour we call mental health difficulties. The dominant discourse is currently one in which these experiences are viewed as pathological and treated as an individual problem. I propose that there is an alternative discourse, such as the one outlined within this book.

We have explored mutual support from many angles, including what it means, and what it can provide for us. We have learnt about mutual support within a developmental context, from both an evolutionary viewpoint and across the human lifespan. We then proceeded to investigate mutual support within the context of mental health; looking at how mutual support can benefit mental health as well as how mental health difficulties can impact on our capacity to connect and interact with others. If we are serious about understanding and treating mental health problems, then it is clear we need a different approach that will provide people with equal opportunities to integrate and engage with the world around them. I believe that the principles underlying mutual support can create this difference and provide a powerful intervention that is capable of making these changes possible. There is now a substantial literature attesting to this, and it is clear that mutual support interventions are both efficacious and effective in reducing mental health difficulties and associated problems. In addition, mutual support interventions are extremely cost-effective, and this is an important factor to consider in the current financial climate, particularly within mental health provision.

The overriding message I wish to give is that all of us have a role to play in bringing about positive change in mental health. I sincerely believe that this change is possible, but it requires each and every one of us to participate – in the way we understand and respond to those experiencing mental health difficulties and in the way we interact with and treat one another.

Further Information

Professional organisations

Association of Therapeutic Communities (ATC)

Founded in 1972, the ATC is the main organisation in the United Kingdom supporting the development of therapeutic communities across different sectors and services (i.e. National Health Service, social services, prison service and voluntary sector). This professional organisation supports the work of therapeutic communities and those that work within them through education and training, research and development and promoting the values of the therapeutic community approach in rehabilitation and recovery.

The ATC website provides essential information about therapeutic communities including a directory that lists member therapeutic communities across the UK and overseas.

Association of Therapeutic Communities
Barns Centre
Church Lane
Toddington
Gloucestershire GL54 4DQ
Tel: 01242 620 077
Website: www.therapeuticcommunities.org

Centre for Community Mental Health (CCMH)

The CCMH is part of the Faculty of Health at Birmingham City University. It works to improve services and life opportunities for people with severe and enduring mental health problems. The Centre concentrates on tackling social exclusion and the development of innovative approaches to service provision through training, education and research.

Centre for Community Mental Health
Birmingham City University
Faculty of Health, City South Campus
Westbourne Road
Edgbaston
Birmingham B15 3TN
Tel: 0121 331 7151
Website: www.health.bcu.ac.uk/ccmh

Charterhouse Group

This organisation was established in 1989 and now operates as a charity that supports, represents, develops and promotes specialist therapeutic childcare in the UK. It is a membership organisation and its members are all providers of specialist residential therapeutic care to children and young people.

Patrick Webb O.B.E.
The Old Farm House
Church Lane, Strubby
Alford
Lincolnshire LN13 0LR
Tel: 01507 451217
Website: www.charterhousegroup.org.uk

Community of Communities (C of C)

The Community of Communities Quality Network (C of C) is a standards-based quality improvement network founded in 2002. The overall aim of C of C is to enable therapeutic communities to evaluate and improve their services by employing methods that reflect their philosophy. To date two-thirds of the UK's therapeutic communities belong to C of C.

Community of Communities
Royal College of Psychiatrists'
Centre for Quality Improvement
4th Floor, Standon House
21 Mansell Street
London E1 8AA
Tel: 020 7977 6697
Website: www.rcpsych.ac.uk/clinicalservicestandards/centreforqualityimprovement/communityofcommunities.aspx

European Federation of Therapeutic Communities (EFTC)

Founded in 1978 and formalised in 1981 on the initiative of a group of therapeutic communities for residential drug treatment, the EFTC is a European federative organisation supporting the psychopedagogical approach helping drug addicts to return to a drug-free life style and to become contributing members of the wider community. Today the EFTC is spread across Europe in 25 countries and represents more than 40 treatment organisations.

European Federation of Therapeutic Communities
Secretary/Treasurer: Mr. Dirk Vandevelde
c/o: T.G. De Kiem
Vluchtenboerstraat 7a
9890 Gavere
Belgium
Tel: + 32 (0) 9 389 6666
Website: www.eftc-europe.com

Institute of Group Analysis (IGA)

Founded in 1971 by S.H. Foulkes and a group of colleagues to provide clinical training in group analytic psychotherapy. The IGA also works with organisations, teams and staff groups as well as offering clinical supervision. A list of accredited group psychotherapists within the UK is provided on its website.

Institute of Group Analysis
1 Daleham Gardens
London NW3 5BY
Tel: 020 7431 2693
Website: www.groupanalysis.org

Planned Environment Therapy Trust (PETT)

A charitable trust established in 1966 to promote effective treatment for children and adults with emotional and psychological disorders. It encourages research, discussion and training in a variety of therapeutic approaches, particularly those known as therapeutic communities. Since it was founded, PETT has produced publications, run conferences and provided grants to individuals for training or research projects in planned environment therapy.

In 1989 the PETT Archive was founded as a resource for interested students and professionals. It is home to a unique and expanding collection of both published and unpublished material relating to environment therapy, milieu therapy and therapeutic communities, from the early work and onwards. It is open to students, historians and researchers. In 2003 the Trust created the Barns Conference and Study Centre. This is also home to the administrative offices for the ATC.

Planned Environment Therapy Trust
Church Lane
Toddington, Cheltenham
Gloucestershire GL54 5DQ
Tel: 01242 621 200
Website: pettrust.org.uk

Therapeutic Communities of America (TCA)

Founded in 1975, TCA is a non-profit membership association for therapeutic communities across the US and Canada.

Therapeutic Communities of America
1601 Connecticut Avenue, Suite 803
Washington DC 20009
USA
Website: www.therapeuticcommunitiesofamerica.org

World Federation of Therapeutic Communities (WFTC)

Founded in 1980, the World Federation of Therapeutic Communities (WFTC) states as its purpose, 'to join together in a worldwide association of sharing, understanding and cooperation within the global TC movement, as well as to widen recognition and acceptance of the Therapeutic Community and the Therapeutic Community approach among health organisations and health delivery systems of international and national bodies'. Their website includes details of a number of regional federations in various parts of the world including Australasia, Asia and South America.

World Federation of Therapeutic Communities, Inc.
54 West 40th Street
New York, NY 10018
USA
Website: www.wftc.org

Adult democratic therapeutic communities

Acorn Programme at The Retreat
The Retreat
Heslington Road
York YO10 5BN
Tel: 01904 412 551
Website: www.theretreatyork.org.uk

The Arbours Association
6 Church Lane
London N8 7BU
Tel: 020 8340 7646
Website: www.arboursassociation.org

Brenchley Unit
The Courtyard
Pudding Lane
Maidstone
Kent ME14 1PA
Tel: 01622 776330
Website: www.kmpt.nhs.uk/personality-disorders-service.htm

Cassel Hospital
1 Ham Common
Richmond
Surrey TM10 7JF
Tel: 020 8483 2900
Website: www.wlmht.nhs.uk/cs/the-cassel

The Cawley Centre
The Maudsley Hospital
Denmark Hill
London SE5 8AZ
Tel: 020 7919 2679
Website: www.slam.nhs.uk

Christ Church Deal
3 Stanhope Road
Deal
Kent CT14 6AB
Tel: 01304 366 512
Website: www.ccd.xpha.net

Community Housing and Therapy
24/5–6 The Coda Centre
189 Munster Road
London SW6 6AW
Tel: 020 7381 5888
Freephone: 0800 018 1261
Website: www.cht.org.uk

Community Housing and Therapy – Dainton House
1a Upper Brighton Road
Surbiton
Surrey KT6 6LQ
Tel: 020 8390 0545

Community Housing and Therapy – Home Base
158 Du Cane Road
London W12 0TX
Tel: 020 8749 4885

Community Housing and Therapy – Lexham House
28 St Charles Square
North Kensington
London W10 6EE
Tel: 020 8969 8745

Community Housing and Therapy – Mount Lodge
5 Upper Avenue
Eastbourne
East Sussex BN21 3UY
Tel: 01323 411 312

Complex Needs Service – Aylesbury
Tindal Centre
Bierton Road, Aylesbury
Buckinghamshire HP20 1HU
Tel: 01296 504 379
Website: www.obmh.nhs.uk/services/specialist/complex-needs

Complex Needs Service – Oxford
Manzil Way
Oxford OX4 1XE
Tel: 01865 455 815
Website: www.psox.org/ocns

Connect
19–21 Park Road
Moseley
Birmingham B13 8AB
Tel: 0121 449 2204
Website: www.connecttc.org

Cumbria Therapeutic Community
Department of Psychotherapy
Beech Lodge
Carleton Clinic
Cumwhinton Drive
Carlisle CA1 3SX
Tel: 01228 603 134
Website: www.cumbriapartnership.nhs.uk/the-itinerant-therapeutic-community.htm

Denbridge House
2 Wells Road
Bickley
Kent BR1 2AJ
Tel: 020 3228 8700
Website: www.slam.nhs.uk

Francis Dixon Lodge
Gipsy Lane
Leicester
Leicestershire LE5 0TD
Tel: 0116 225 6800
Website: www.leicspt.nhs.uk

Garden Villa
Psychotherapy Department
Upper Garden Villa
Aberdeen AB25 2ZH
Tel: 01224 557 321

The Haven Project
1 Glen Avenue
Lexden
Colchester
Essex CO3 3RP
Tel: 01206 287 316 (9–5pm)
Tel: 01206 572 215 (24-hour crisis line)
Website: www.thehavenproject.org.uk

Lothlorien
Corsock
Castle Douglas
Dumfries & Galloway DG7 3DR
Tel: 01644 440 602
Website: www.lothlorien.tc

Mandala Therapeutic Community
Mandala Centre
Gregory Boulevard
Forest Fields
Nottingham NG7 6LB
Tel: 0115 960 2820
Website: www.nottinghamshirehealthcare.nhs.uk

Philadelphia Association
4 Marty's Yard
17 Hampstead High Street
London NW3 1QW
Tel: 020 7794 2652
Website: www.philadelphia-association.co.uk

Red House Psychotherapy Service
78 Manchester Road
Swinton
Manchester M27 5FG
Tel: 0161 794 0875
Website: www.gmw.nhs.uk

Richmond Fellowship – Pele Tower
3 Elms West
Ashbrook
Sunderland SR2 7LU
Tel: 0191 565 8111
Website: www.peletower.org.uk

Therapeutic Communities Services North – Diverse Pathways
Tuke House
60 Sholebroke Avenue
Leeds LS7 3HB
Tel: 0161 708 2800

Threshold
432 Antrim Road
Belfast BT15 5GB
Northern Ireland
Tel: 028 9087 1313
Website: www.threshold-services.co.uk

Threshold Services – Chikara
9-11 Belgravia Avenue
Belfast B79 7BJ
Northern Ireland
Tel: 028 9066 8302

Threshold Services – Glencarn House
79 Somerton Road
Glengormley BT15 4DG
Northern Ireland
Tel: 028 9087 9191

Threshold Services – Kharaminn House
2 Eglington Lane
Portrush
Northern Ireland
Tel: 028 7082 1111

Winterbourne House
53–55 Argyle Road
Reading
Berkshire RG1 7YL
Tel: 0118 956 1250
Website: www.berkshirehealthcare.nhs.uk

Adult democratic therapeutic communities for offenders

HMP Blundeston
Therapeutic Community HMP Blundeston
Lowestoft
Suffolk NR32 5BG
Tel: 01502 734 664
Website: www.hmprisonservice.gov.uk

HMP Dovegate Assessment Unit
ARU Therapeutic Community
HMP Dovegate
Uttoxeter
Staffordshire ST14 8XR
Tel: 01283 829 547
Website: www.hmprisonservice.gov.uk

HMP Dovegate – Avalon TC
Avalon Therapeutic Community
HMP Dovegate
Uttoxeter
Staffordshire ST14 8XR
Tel: 01283 829 575
Website: www.hmprisonservice.gov.uk

HMP Dovegate – Camelot Therapeutic Community
Camelot Therapeutic Community
HMP Dovegate
Uttoxeter
Staffordshire ST14 8XR
Tel: 01283 829 527
Website: www.hmprisonservice.gov.uk

HMP Dovegate – Endeavour Therapeutic Community
Endeavour Therapeutic Community
HMP Dovegate
Uttoxeter
Staffordshire ST14 8XR
Tel: 01283 829 570
Website: www.hmprisonservice.gov.uk

HMP Dovegate – Genesis Therapeutic Community
Genesis Therapeutic Community
HMP Dovegate
Uttoxeter
Staffordshire ST14 8XR
Tel: 01283 829 532
Website: www.hmprisonservice.gov.uk

HMP Gartree
Gartree Therapeutic Community
Gallowfield Road
Market Harborough
Leicestershire LE16 7RP
Tel: 01858 436 600 ext 6789
Website: www.hmprisonservice.gov.uk

HMP Grendon Assessment Unit
Grendon Underwood
Aylesbury
Buckinghamshire HP18 0TL
Tel: 01296 443 167
Website: www.hmprisonservice.gov.uk

HMP Grendon A
Grendon Underwood
Aylesbury
Buckinghamshire HP18 0TL
Tel: 01296 443 122
Website: www.hmprisonservice.gov.uk

HMP Grendon B
Grendon Underwood
Aylesbury
Buckinghamshire HP18 0TL
Tel: 01296 443 241
Website: www.hmprisonservice.gov.uk

HMP Grendon C
Grendon Underwood
Aylesbury
Buckinghamshire HP18 0TL
Tel: 01296 443 130
Website: www.hmprisonservice.gov.uk

HMP Grendon G
Grendon Underwood
Aylesbury
Buckinghamshire HP18 0TL
Tel: 01296 443 141
Website: www.hmprisonservice.gov.uk

HMP Send
Ripley Road
Woking
Surrey GU23 7LJ
Tel: 01483 471 264
Website: www.hmprisonservice.gov.uk

Millfields Medium Secure Unit
Forensic Personality Disorder Services
John Howard Centre
12 Kenworthy Road
Homerton
London E9 5TD
Tel: 020 8510 2003/5/6
Website: www.eastlondon.nhs.uk

Addiction therapeutic communities

Coolmine TC – Ashleigh House
Coolmine House
19 Lord Edward Street
Dublin 2
Ireland
Tel: +35 31 825 1100
Website: www.coolmine.ie

Coolmine TC – The Lodge
Coolmine House
19 Lord Edward Street
Dublin 2
Ireland
Tel: +35 31 821 4545
Website: www.coolmine.ie

Ley Community
Sandy Croft
Sandy Lane
Yarnton
Oxfordshire OX5 1PB
Tel: 01865 378600
Website: www.ley.co.uk

Phoenix Futures – Sheffield
Storth Oaks
229 Graham Road
Ranmoor
Sheffield S10 3GS
Tel: 0114 230 8230
Website: www.phoenix-futures.org.uk

Phoenix Futures – Tyneside
Westoe Drive
South Shields
Tyne and Wear NE33 3EW
Tel: 0191 454 5544
Website: www.phoenix-futures.org.uk

Sefton Park
Residential Alcohol & Drugs Rehabilitation Centre
& Therapeutic Community
10 Royal Crescent
Weston-super-Mare
Somerset BS23 2AX
Tel: 01934 626 371
Website: www.sefton-park.com

Addiction therapeutic communities for offenders

HMP Channings Wood
Denbury
Newton Abbot
Devon TQ12 6DW
Tel: 01803 814 600
Website: www.hmprisonservice.gov.uk

HMP Garth
Ulnes Walton Lane
Leyland
Preston PR26 8NE
Tel: 01772 443 300
Website: www.hmprisonservice.gov.uk

HMP Holme House
Holme House Road
Stockton on Tees TS18 2QU
Tel: 01642 744 000
Website: www.hmprisonservice.gov.uk

HMP Wymott
Ulnes Walton Lane
Leyland
Preston PR26 8LW
Tel: 01772 442 000
Website: www.hmprisonservice.gov.uk

Therapeutic communities for children and young people

Amberleigh Residential Therapeutic School
Welshpool
Powys
Wales
Tel: 01938 554 111
Website: www.amberleighcare.co.uk

Amicus Community
PO Box 79
Arundel
West Sussex BN18 9XA
Tel: 01903 885 135
Website: www.theamicuscommunity.com

Ankea House
20 Ash Street
Southport PR9 9BY
Tel: 01704 547326
Website: www.ankeahouse.co.uk

Barford Care and Therapy Services – Willow Lodge
Sapcote Road
Stoney Stanton
Leicestershire LE9 4DW
Tel: 01455 617 070
Website: www.barfordcare.com

Benjamin UK Ltd
Ascott Lodge
Lower Ascott
Wing LU7 0PU
Tel: 0800 092 1312
Website: www.benjaminuk.co.uk

Bryn Melyn Care
2 High Street
Dawley
Telford TF4 2ET
Tel: 01952 504 715
Website: www.brynmelyncare.com

Donyland Lodge
Fingringhoe Road
Rowhedge
Colchester
Essex CO5 7JL
Tel: 01206 728 869
Website: www.donyland.org.uk

Ferndearle Child Care Services
13 Highpoint Business Village
Henwood
Ashford
Kent TN24 8DH
Tel: 01622 880 676
Website: www.ferndearle.com

Friends Therapeutic Community – Glebe House
Shudy Camps
Cambridge CB21 4QH
Tel: 01799 584 359
Website: www.glebehouse.org.uk

Ingleside Children's Home Ltd
3 Mayfield Road
Sanderstead
Surrey CR2 0BG
Tel: 020 8405 6777
Website: www.ingleside.co.uk

Lioncare Group
The Lioncare Group
Lioncare House
58a Livingstone Road
Hove BN3 3WL
Tel: 01273 720 424
Website: www.lioncare.co.uk

Little Acorns
London Beach Farm
Ashford Road
St Michaels
Tenterden
Kent TN30 6SR
Tel: 01233 850 422
Website: www.choicelifestyles.net

Mulberry Bush School
Abingdon Road
Standlake
Witney
Oxfordshire OX29 7RW
Tel: 01865 300 202
Website: www.mulberrybush.org.uk

Oasis Young People's Care Services
PO Box 5597
Southend-on-Sea
Essex SS0 7WE
Tel: 01702 555 055
Website: www.oasisypcs.com

Oracle Care Ltd
Unit 2
Dane Valley Mill
Havannah Street
Congleton CW12 2AH
Tel: 0870 850 2949
Website: www.oraclecare.com

Quality Protects Children Ltd
Hill House
Archway Road
Huyton L36 9XB
Tel: 0151 949 5690
Website: www.qpconline.co.uk

RAAC Care
23 Mulford Hill
Tadley
Hampshire RG23 3LQ
Tel: 0118 933 3440
Website: www.raacltd.co.uk

Richmond Psychosocial Foundation International – Lytton House
27 Lytton Grove
London SW15 2EZ
Tel: 020 8788 1944
Website: www.rpfi.org

The Roaches Independent School
Upper School
Tunstall Road
Knypersley
Stoke-on-Trent ST8 7AB
Tel: 01782 523 479/516 207
Website: www.roachesschool.co.uk

The Roaches Independent School
Lower School
Lower Roach End
Meerbrook
Nr Leek
Staffordshire ST13 8TA
Tel: 01298 79989
Website: www.roachesschool.co.uk

Roundhouse Care – The Hedgerows
467 Rawnsley Road
Hednesford
Cannock WS12 1RB
Tel: 01543 871 464
Website: www.roundhousecare.org

Smyly Trust Services
15 Rock Hill
Blackrock
Co. Dublin
Ireland
Tel: +35 31 283 2071
Website: www.smylytrust.ie

Tregynon Hall School (SENAD group)
Cefngwyddfod
Tregynon
Newtown SY16 3PG
Tel: 01686 650 330
Website: www.tregynonhall.com

TulipCare Group
19–20 Bourne Court
Southend Road
Woodford Green IG8 8HD
Tel: 0845 094 3550
Website: www.tulipcare.co.uk

Tumblewood Community School
The Laurels
Westbury
Wiltshire BA13 4LF
Tel: 01373 824 466
Website: www.tumblewoodcommunity.org.uk

Willowgrove House Special School
1–6 Willowgrove
Craigshill
Livingston
West Lothian EH54 5LU
Tel: 01506 434 274

Therapeutic communities for people with learning disabilities

Camphill Advisory Service
19 South Road
Stourbridge DY8 3YA
Tel: 01384 441 680
Website: www.camphill.org.uk

Camphill – Albion House, Grange Village
Newham-on-Severn
Gloucestershire GL14 1HJ
Tel: 01594 516 246

Camphill – Botton Village
Danby
Whitby YO21 2NJ
Tel: 01287 661 300

Camphill – Delrow House, St Albans
Hilfield Lane
Aldenham
Hertfordshire WD25 8DJ
Tel: 01923 856 006

Camphill – East Anglia
Thornage Hall
Thornage
Holt NR25 7QH
Tel: 01263 860 305

Camphill – Larchfield Community
Stokesley Road
Hemlington
Middlesbrough TS8 9DY
Tel: 01642 579 800

Camphill – Milton Keynes Community
Japonica Lane
Willen Park
Milton Keynes MK15 9JY
Tel: 01908 235 000

Pennine Camphill Community
Wood Lane
Chapelthorpe
Wakefield WF4 3JL
Tel: 01924 255 281

Mutual support groups and organisations

Al-Anon Family Groups UK and Eire (for families and friends of alcoholics)
61 Great Dover Street
London SE1 4YF
Tel: 020 7403 0888
Website: www.al-anonuk.org.uk

Alcoholics Anonymous
PO Box 1
10 Toft Green
York YO1 7NJ
National Helpline: 0845 769 7555
Website: www.alcoholics-anonymous.org.uk

Anxiety UK
Zion Community Resource Centre
339 Stretford Road
Hulme
Manchester M15 4ZY
Tel: 0844 477 5774
Website: www.anxietyuk.org.uk

Beating Eating Disorders (BEAT)
103 Prince of Wales Road
Norwich NR1 1DW
Tel: 0845 634 1414
Website: www.b-eat.co.uk

Carers UK
20 Great Dover Street
London SE1 4LX
Tel: 020 7378 4999
Website: www.carersuk.org

Cruse Bereavement Care
PO Box 800
Richmond
Surrey TW9 1RG
Tel: 0844 477 9400
Website: www.crusebereavementcare.org.uk

Depression Alliance
Suite 212, Spitfire Studios
63–71 Collier Street
London N1 9BE
Tel: 0845 123 2320
Website: www.depressionalliance.org

Emergence (service-user led organisation with the aim of supporting people affected by difficulties associated with personality disorder)
London House
271–273 King Street
London W6 9LX
Tel: 020 8233 2854/2855
Website: www.emergenceplus.org.uk

Families Anonymous (self-help organisation for family and friends of drug users)
Doddington and Rollo Community Association
Charlotte Despard Avenue
Battersea
London SW11 5HD
Tel: 0845 120 0660
Website: www.famanon.org.uk

Hearing Voices Network
79 Lever Street
Manchester M1 1FL
Tel: 0845 122 8641
Website: www.hearing-voices.org

National Association for People Abused in Childhood (NAPAC)
42 Curtain Road
London EC2A 3NH
Tel: 0800 085 3330
Website: www.napac.org.uk

OCD-UK (Obsessive Compulsive Disorder)
PO Box 8955
Nottingham
NG10 9AU
Tel: 0845 120 3778
Website: www.ocduk.org

Rethink (for everyone affected by severe mental health problems)
89 Albert Embankment
London SE1 7TP
Tel: 0845 456 0455
Website: www.rethink.org

UK Narcotics Anonymous
Tel: 0300 999 1212
Website: www.ukna.org

Other useful contacts

Asylum
Website: www.asylumonline.net

Coming Off Psychiatric Medication
Website: www.comingoff.com

Community Psychology Network UK
Website: www.compsy.org.uk

Mental Health America (MHA)
Website: www.mentalhealthamerica.net

MIND
Tel: 0845 766 0163
Website: www.mind.org.uk

Patient UK
Website: www.patient.co.uk

Psychminded
Website: www.psychminded.co.uk

Soteria Network
Website: www.soterianetwork.org.uk

Therapeutic Community Open Forum (TC-OF)
Website: www.tc-of.org.uk

References

Ainsworth, M.D.S., Blehar, M.C., Waters, E. and Wall, S. (1978) *Patterns of Attachment.* Hillsdale, NJ: Erlbaum.

Albee, G.W. (1982) 'Preventing psychopathology and promoting human potential.' *American Psychologist 37,* 9, 1043–1050.

Barker, C. and Pistrang, N. (2002) 'Psychotherapy and social support: Integrating research on psychological helping.' *Clinical Psychology Review 22,* 361–379.

Barker, C., Pistrang, N., Shapiro, D.A. and Shaw, I. (1990) 'Coping and help-seeking in the UK adult population.' *British Journal of Clinical Psychology 29,* 271–285.

Barrera, M. (1986) 'Distinctions between social support concepts, measures, and models.' *American Journal of Community Psychology 14,* 413–445.

Barrett, L., Dunbar, R. and Lycett, J. (2001) *Human Evolutionary Psychology.* London: Palgrave Macmillan.

Bartholomew, K. and Horowitz, L.M. (1991) 'Attachment styles among young adults: A test of a four-category model.' *Journal of Personality and Social Psychology 61,* 226–244.

Bebbington, P.E., Brugha, T.S., Meltzer, H., Jenkins, R., Ceresa, C., Farrell, M. and Lewis, G. (2000) 'Neurotic disorders and the receipt of psychiatric treatment.' *Psychological Medicine 30,* 1369–1376.

Berke, J.H., Masoliver, C. and Ryan, T. (eds) (1995) *Sanctuary: The Arbours Experience of Alternative Community Care.* London: Process Press.

Biggs, V. (1987) 'The In-patients' Views of the Cassel Experience.' In R. Kennedy, A. Heymans and L. Tishler (eds) *The Family as In-Patient: Families and Adolescents at the Cassel Hospital.* London: Free Association Books.

Bion, W.R. (1960) *Experiences in Groups.* London: Tavistock Publications.

Bloom, J.R. (1990) 'The relationship of social support and health.' *Social Science and Medicine 30,* 635–637.

Borkman, T.J. (1990) 'Experiential, Professional and Lay Frames of Reference.' In T.J. Powell (ed) *Working with Self-Help.* Silver Spring, MD: NASW Press.

Bowlby, J. (1969) *Attachment and Loss, Vol. 1, Attachment.* London: Hogarth Press.

Bowlby, J. (1973) *Attachment and Loss, Vol. 2, Separation: Anxiety and Anger.* London: Hogarth Press.

Bowlby, J. (1979) *The Making and Breaking of Affectional Bonds.* London: Tavistock.

Bowlby, J. (1980) *Attachment and Loss, Vol. 3, Loss: Sadness and Depression.* London: Hogarth Press.

Broekaert, E., Kooyman, M. and Ottenberg, D. (1998) 'The "new" drug-free therapeutic community. Challenging encounter of classic and open therapeutic communities.' *Journal of Substance Abuse Treatment 15,* 595–597.

Brown, L.D., Shepherd, M.D., Merkle, E.C., Wituk, S.A. and Meissen, G. (2008) 'Understanding how participation in a consumer-run organization relates to recovery.' *American Journal of Community Psychology 42,* 167–178.

Carlson, E.A., Sroufe, L.A. and Egeland, B. (2004) 'The construction of experience: A longitudinal study of representation and behavior.' *Child Development 75,* 66–83.

Cassel, J. (1976) 'The contribution of the social environment to host resistance.' *American Journal of Epidemiology 104,* 107–123.

Chazan, R. (2001) *The Group as Therapist.* London: Jessica Kingsley Publishers.

Chien, W.T., Thompson, D.R. and Norman, I. (2008) 'Evaluation of a peer-led mutual support group for Chinese families of people with schizophrenia.' *American Journal of Community Psychology 42,* 122–134.

Clark, D.H. (1965) 'The therapeutic community – concept, practice and future.' *British Journal of Psychiatry 111,* 947–954.

Coates, D. and Winston, T. (1983) 'Counteracting the deviance of depression: Peer support groups for victims.' *Journal of Social Issues 39,* 169–194.

Cobb, S. (1976) 'Social support as a moderator of life stress.' *Psychosomatic Medicine 38,* 300–314.

Cohen, S. and Wills, T.A. (1985) 'Stress, social support, and the buffering process.' *Psychological Bulletin 98,* 310–357.

Cook, J.A., Heller, T. and Pickett-Schenk, S.A. (1999) 'The effect of support group participation on caregiver burden among parents of adult offspring with severe mental illness.' *Family Relations 48,* 405–410.

Corrigan, P.W. and Penn, D.L. (1999) 'Lessons from social psychology on discrediting psychiatric stigma.' *American Psychologist 54,* 765–776.

Cowen, E.L. (1982) 'Help is where you find it: Four informal helping groups.' *American Psychologist 37,* 385–395.

Cross, D.G., Sheehan, P.W. and Kahn, J.A. (1980) 'Alternative advice and counsel in psychotherapy.' *Journal of Consulting and Clinical Psychology 48,* 615–625.

Cutrona, C.E. (1990) 'Stress and social support: In search of optimal matching.' *Journal of Social and Clinical Psychology 9,* 3–14.

Cutrona, C.E. (1996) *Social Support in Couples.* Thousand Oaks, CA: Sage.

Davies, S., Campling, P. and Ryan, K. (1999) 'Therapeutic community provision at regional and district levels.' *The Psychiatrist 23,* 79–83.

Davison, K.P., Pennebaker, H.W. and Dickerson, S.S. (2000). 'Who talks? The social psychology of illness support groups.' *American Psychologist 55,* 2, 205–217.

De Leon, G. (2000) *The Therapeutic Community Theory, Model and Method.* New York, NY: Springer.

Dermatis, H., Salke, M., Galanter, M. and Bunt, G. (2001) 'The role of social cohesion among residents in a therapeutic community.' *Journal of Substance Abuse Treatment 21*, 105–110.

Dietrich, D. (2006) 'Psychological health of young adults who experienced early parent death: MMPI trends.' *Journal of Clinical Psychology 40*, 4, 901–908.

Dolan, B.M., Warren, F.M., Menzies, D. and Norton, K. (1996) 'Cost offset following specialist treatment of severe personality disorders.' *Psychiatric Bulletin 20*, 413–417.

Dooley, D. (1985) 'Causal Inference in the Study of Social Support.' In S. Cohen and S.L. Syme (eds) *Social Support and Health*. New York, NY: Academic Press.

Dozier, M., Stovall, K.C. and Albus, K.E. (1999) 'Attachment and Psychopathology in Adulthood.' In J. Cassidy and P.R. Shaver (eds) *Handbook of Attachment: Theory, Research and Clinical Implications*. London: Guilford Press.

Drahorad, C. with Frances and Sue (1999) 'Reflections on being a patient in a therapeutic community.' *Therapeutic Communities 20*, 3, 195–215.

Dunkel-Schetter, C. (1984) 'Social support and cancer: Findings based on patient interviews and their implications.' *Journal of Social Issues 40*, 77–98.

Dunkel-Schetter, C. and Bennett, T.L. (1990) 'Differentiating the Cognitive and Behavioral Aspects of Social Support.' In B.R. Sarason, I.G. Sarason and G.R. Pierce (eds) *Social Support: An Interactional View*. New York, NY: Wiley.

Edmunson, E.D., Bedell, J.R., Archer, R.P. and Gordon, R.E. (1982) 'Integrating Skill Building and Peer Support in Mental Health Treatment: The Early Intervention and Community Network Development Projects.' In A.M. Jeger and R.S. Slotnick (eds) *Community Mental Health and Behavioral Ecology*. New York, NY: Plenum Press.

Erikson, E. (1968) *Identity: Youth and Crisis*. London: Faber.

Festinger, L. (1954) 'A theory of social comparison processes.' *Human Relations 7*, 117–140.

Foulkes, S.R. (1948) *Introduction to Group Analytic Psychotherapy*. London: Heinemann.

Fromm, E. (1956) *The Sane Society*. London: Routledge and Kegan Paul.

Galanter, M. (1988) 'Zealous self-help groups as adjuncts to psychiatric treatment: A study of Recovery Inc.' *American Journal of Psychiatry 145*, 10, 1248–1253.

Glatt, M.M. (1985, November) 'The Wormwood Scrubs Annexe: Reflections on the Working and Functioning of an Addicts' Therapeutic Community within a Prison.' *Prison Care*.

Goldberg, D. and Huxley, P. (1992) *Common Mental Disorders: A Bio-Social Model*. London: Routledge.

Goldstrom, I.D., Campbell, J., Rogers, J.A., Lambert, D.B., Blacklow, B., Henderson, M.J. and Manderscheid, R.W. (2006). 'National estimates for mental health mutual support groups, self-help organizations, and consumer-operated services.' *Administration and Policy in Mental Health and Mental Health Services Research 33*, 92–103.

Grant, C., Goodenough, T., Harvey, I. and Hine, C. (2000) 'A randomised controlled trial and economic evaluation of a referrals facilitator between primary care and the voluntary sector.' *British Medical Journal 320*, 419–423.

Haaga, D.A.F. (2000) 'Introduction to the special section on stepped care models in psychotherapy.' *Journal of Consulting and Clinical Psychology 68*, 547–548.

Haigh, R. (2002) 'Therapeutic community research: Past, present and future.' *Psychiatric Bulletin 26*, 65–68.

Haigh, R., Kennard, D., Lees, J. and Morris, M. (2002, March) 'The foreword to the final revised version of the therapeutic community standards, which form the basis for the quality network mutual audit exercise.' *The Joint Newsletter of the Association of Therapeutic Communities, the Charterhouse Group of Therapeutic Communities, and the Planned Environment Therapy Trust.* No. 4, p.13.

Haigh, R. and Lees, J. (2008) '"Fusion TCs": Divergent histories, converging challenges.' *Therapeutic Communities 29*, 4, 347–374.

Helgeson, V.S. and Cohen, S. (1996) 'Social support and adjustment to cancer: Reconciling descriptive, correlational, and intervention research.' *Health Psychology 15*, 135–148.

Helgeson, V.S. and Gottlieb, B.H. (2000) 'Support Groups.' In S. Cohen, I.G. Underwood and B.H. Gottlieb (eds) *Social Support Measurement and Intervention: A Guide for Health and Social Scientists.* Oxford: Oxford University Press.

Helgeson, V.S. and Mickelson, K.D. (1995). 'Motives for social comparison.' *Personality and Social Psychology Bulletin 21*, 1200–1209.

Hogan, B., Linden, W. and Najarian, B. (2002) 'Social support interventions: Do they work?' *Clinical Psychology Review 22*, 381–440.

Horowitz, L.M. (1979) 'On the cognitive structure of interpersonal problems treated in psychotherapy.' *Journal of Consulting and Clinical Psychology 47*, 5–15.

House, J., Landis, S.A. and Umberson, D. (1988) 'Social relationships and health.' *Science 241*, 540–545.

Humphreys, K. and Rappaport, J. (1994) 'Researching self-help/mutual aid groups and organizations: Many roads, one journey.' *Applied and Preventative Psychology 3*, 217–231.

Jablensky, A., Sartorius, N., Ernberg, G., Anker, M., Korten, A., Cooper, J.E., Day, R. and Bertelsen, A. (1992) 'Schizophrenia: Manifestations, incidence and course in different cultures. A World Health Organization ten-country study.' *Psychological Medicine Monograph Supplement 20*, 1–97.

Jacobs, M.K. and Goodman, G. (1989) 'Psychology and self-help groups: Predictions on a partnership.' *American Psychologist 44*, 3, 536–545.

Jones, M. (1968) *Social Psychiatry in Practice.* Harmondsworth: Penguin.

Jones, M. (1979) 'The Therapeutic Community, Social Learning and Social Change.' In R.D. Hinshelwood and N. Manning (eds) *Therapeutic Communities: Reflections and Progress.* London: Routledge and Kegan Paul.

Katz, A. and Bender, E. (1976) *Self-help groups in the Modern World.* New York, NY: New Viewpoints.

Kelly, J.F., Stout, R., Zywiak, W. and Schneider, R. (2006) 'A 3-year study of addiction mutual-help group participation following intensive outpatient treatment.' *Alcoholism: Clinical and Experimental Research 30*, 8, 1381–1392.

Kennard, D. (2000) *An Introduction to Therapeutic Communities*. London: Jessica Kingsley Publishers.

Kennard, D. (2004) 'The therapeutic community as an adaptive treatment modality across different settings.' *Psychiatric Quarterly 75*, 3, 295–307.

Kessler, R.C., Mickelson, K.D. and Zhao, S. (1997) 'Patterns and correlates of self-help group membership in the United States.' *Social Policy 27*, 27–46.

Kropotkin, P. (1972) *Mutual Aid: A Factor of Evolution*. New York, NY: University Press. (Original work published in 1902)

Kurtz, L.F. (1988) 'Mutual aid for affective disorders: The manic depressive and depressive association.' *American Journal of Orthopsychiatry 58*, 1, 152–155.

Kyrouz, E., Humphreys, K. and Loomis, C. (2002) 'A Review of Research on the Effectiveness of Self-Help Mutual Aid Groups.' In B.J. White and E.J. Madara (eds) *The Self-Help Sourcebook: Your Guide to Community and Online Support Groups* (7th edn). Denville, NJ: American Self-Help Group Clearinghouse.

Laing, R.D. (1967) *The Politics of Experience and the Bird of Paradise*. Harmondsworth: Penguin.

Lazarus, R.S. (1975) 'A cognitively oriented psychologist looks at biofeedback.' *American Psychologist 30*, 553–561.

Lees, J., Manning, N. and Rawlings, B. (1999). *Therapeutic Community Effectiveness: A Systematic International Review of Therapeutic Treatment for People with Personality Disorders and Mentally Disordered Offenders*. CRD Report 17. York: NHS Centre for Reviews and Dissemination, University of York.

Lees, J., Manning, N. and Rawlings, B. (2004). 'A culture of enquiry: Research evidence and the therapeutic community.' *Psychiatric Quarterly 75*, 3, 279–294.

Lieberman, M.A. (1993) 'Self-help Groups.' In H.I. Kaplan and B.J. Sadock (eds) *Comprehensive Group Psychotherapy*. Baltimore, MD: Williams & Wilkins.

Lloyd, C. (1980) 'Life events and depressive disorder reviewed. I. Events as predisposing factors.' *Archives of General Psychiatry 37*, 5, 529–535.

Loat, M. (2006) 'Sharing the struggle: An exploration of mutual support processes in a therapeutic community.' *International Journal of Therapeutic Communities 27*, 2, 211–228.

Lyons, J.S., Perotta, P. and Hancher-Kvam, S. (1988) 'Perceived social support from family and friends: Measurement across disparate samples.' *Journal of Personality Assessment 52*, 1, 42–47.

Main, M. and Solomon, J. (1990) 'Procedures for Identifying Infants as Disorganized/Disoriented During the Ainsworth Strange Situation.' In M.T. Greenberg, D. Cicchetti and E.M. Cummings (eds) *Attachment in the Preschool Years: Theory, Research and Intervention*. Chicago, IL: University of Chicago Press.

Main, T.F. (1946) 'The hospital as a therapeutic institution.' *Bulletin of the Menninger Clinic 10*, 66–70. (Reprinted in 1996 in *Therapeutic Communities 17*, 2, 77–80)

Mäkikyrö, T., Sauvola, A., Moring, J., Veijola, J., Nieminen, P., Järvelin, M.-R. and Isohanni, M. (1998) 'Hospital-treated psychiatric disorders in adults with a single-parent and two-parent family background: A 28-year follow-up of the 1966 Northern Finland Birth Cohort.' *Family Process 37*, 3, 335–344.

Maton, K.I. (1988) 'Social support, organizational characteristics, psychological well-being and group appraisal in three self-help group populations.' *American Journal of Community Psychology 16*, 53–77.

Mind (2004) *Not Alone? Isolation and Mental Distress*. London: Mind.

Morris, M. (2004) *Dangerous and Severe – Process, Programme and Person: Grendon's Work*. London: Jessica Kingsley Publishers.

NIMHE (2003) *Personality Disorder: No Longer a Diagnosis of Exclusion: Policy Implementation Guidance for the Development of Services for People with Personality Disorder*. London: Department of Health.

Peters-Golden, H. (1982) 'Breast cancer: Varied perceptions of social support in the illness experience.' *Social Science and Medicine 16*, 483–491.

Pines, M. and Schlapobersky, J. (2000) 'Group Methods in Adult Psychiatry.' In M. Gelder (ed.) *New Oxford Textbook of Psychiatry*. Oxford: Oxford University Press.

Pistrang, N., Barker, C. and Humphreys, K. (2008) 'Mutual help groups for mental health problems: A review of effectiveness studies.' *American Journal of Community Psychology 42*, 110–121.

Planned Environment Therapy Trust. Information leaflet. (n.d.) www.otherpeopleschildren.org.uk/documents/pett_flyer_c2002.pdf

Rapoport, R.N. (1960) *Community as Doctor*. London: Tavistock.

Richardson, L. (2002) 'Substance abusers' friendships and social support networks in the therapeutic community.' *Therapeutic Communities 23*, 2, 85–104.

Riessman, F. (1965) 'The helper therapy principle.' *Social Work 10*, 29–38.

Roberts, L.J., Salem, D., Rappaport, J., Toro, P.A., Luke, D.A. and Seidman, E. (1999) 'Giving and receiving help: Interpersonal transactions in mutual-help meetings and psychosocial adjustment of members.' *American Journal of Community Psychology 27*, 841–868.

Robertson, J. and Bowlby, J. (1952) 'Responses of young children to separation from their mothers.' *Courrier of the International Children's Centre, Paris II*, 131–140.

Sarason, B.R., Sarason, I.G. and Pierce, G.R. (eds) (1990) *Social Support: An Interactional View*. New York, NY: Wiley.

Sarason, I.G., Sarason, B.R. and Pierce, G.R. (1990) 'Social support: The search for theory.' *Journal of Social and Clinical Psychology 9*, 133–147.

Sartorius, N., Jablensky, A. and Shapiro, R. (1977) 'Two years follow-up of the patients included in the WHO International Pilot study of schizophrenia.' *Psychological Medicine 7*, 529–541.

Silverman, P. (1985) 'Tertiary/Secondary Prevention – Preventive Intervention: The Case for Mutual Help Groups.' In R.K. Conyne (ed.) *The Group Workers' Handbook*. Springfield, IL: Charles C. Thomas.

Skilton, L. (2007) 'Working Paper: Measuring Societal Wellbeing in the UK.' Newport: Office for National Statistics

Smith, J.A. and Osborn, M. (2003) 'Interpretative Phenomenological Analysis.' In J.A. Smith (ed.) *Qualitative Psychology: A Practical Guide to Research Methods*. London: Sage.

Spiegel, D., Bloom, J.R., Kraemer, H.C. and Gottheil, E. (1989) 'Effect of psychosocial treatment on survival of patients with metastatic breast cancer.' *The Lancet 14*, 888–891.

Taylor, S.E. (2003) *Health Psychology.* New York, NY: McGraw-Hill.

Toro, P.A., Reischl, T.M., Zimmerman, M.A., Rappaport, J., Seidman, E., Luke, D.A. and Roberts, L.J. (1988) 'Professionals in mutual help groups: Impact on social climate and members' behavior.' *Journal of Consulting and Clinical Psychology 56*, 631–632.

Toseland, R.W., Rossiter, C.M. and Labrecque, M.S. (1989) 'The effectiveness of two kinds of support groups for caregivers.' *Social Service Review 63*, 415–432.

Trivedi, P. (2002) 'Racism, Social-Exclusion and Mental Health: A Black Users' Perspective.' In K. Bhui (ed.) *Racism and Mental Health: Prejudice and Suffering.* London: Jessica Kingsley Publishers.

Tuke, S. (1813) *Description of The Retreat.* Republished in 1996. London: Process Books.

Waxler, N.E. (1979) 'Is outcome for schizophrenia better in non-industrial societies: The case for Sri Lanka.' *Journal of Nervous and Mental Disease 167*, 144–158.

White, B.J. and Madara, E.J. (eds) (2002) *The Self-Help Group Sourcebook: Your Guide to Community and Online Support Groups* (7th edn). Denville, NJ: American Self-Help Group Clearinghouse.

Whiteley, J.S. (1999) 'Attachment theory and milieu therapy.' *Group Analytic Contexts 14*, 24–27.

Whiteley, J.S. and Collis, M. (1987) 'The therapeutic factors in group psychotherapy applied to the therapeutic community.' *International Journal of Therapeutic Communities 8*, 1, 21–32.

Willig, C. (2001) *Introducing Qualitative Research in Psychology: Adventures in Theory and Method.* Buckingham: Open University Press.

Wills, W.D. (1945) *The Barns Experiment.* London: Allen & Unwin.

World Health Organization (1979) *An International Follow-Up Study of Schizophrenia.* Chichester: Wiley.

World Health Organization (2001) *The World Health Report 2001 – Mental Health: New Understanding, New Hope.* Geneva: WHO.

Wortman, C.B. and Dunkel-Schetter, C. (1987) 'Conceptual and Methodological Issues in the Study of Social Support.' In A. Baum and J. Singer (eds) *Handbook of Psychology and Health.* Hillsdale, NJ: Lawrence Erlbaum.

Yalom, I.D. (1995) *The Theory and Practice of Group Psychotherapy* (4th edn). New York, NY: Basic Books.

Subject Index

accessing mutual support groups 92–4
activity groups 58, 59
addiction problems
    support models 72
    therapeutic support communities 120–1
adolescence 36
advertising and publicity 96–7
aims and goals (mutual support groups) 95, 98, 99
Al-Anon Family Groups 127
Alcoholics Anonymous (AA) 60, 127
Amberleigh Residential Therapeutic School 122
Amicus Community 122
anonymity 62–3
anti-psychiatry movement 72–3
Anxiety UK 127
Approved Clinicians (AC) 53
Arbours therapeutic community 87, 113
Association of Therapeutic Communities (ATC) 109
attachment styles 26–8
attachment theory 25–32
    across lifespan 28–30
    and mental health 31–2

Beating Eating Disorders (BEAT) 128
Belmont Hospital (Surrey) 70
Bion, Wilfred 69, 86
Bowlby, John 25–32
Brenchley Unit (Kent) 113
Bridget, Harold 69

C of C see Community of Communities (C of C) Quality Network
Camphill communities 126–7
Carers UK 128
Care in the Community 40–1, 103–4
Cassel Hospital (Richmond) 70, 87–8, 113
Cawley Centre (London) 113
Centre for Community Mental Health (CCMH) 109–10
change agents (group therapy) 56–8
Charterhouse Group 110
children and young adults, therapeutic communities 122–6
Clark, David 70–71

Community of Communities (C of C) Quality Network 74–7, 110
Community Treatment Orders (CTOs) 105
Community-based care policies 40–1, 103–4
Complex Needs Services 114
confidentiality issues 98
Cooper, David 72
Cruse Bereavement Care 128

definitions of mutual support 18–19
'democratic therapeutic community' 71
Denbridge House (Kent) 115
Depression Alliance 128
development stages see psychosocial stages of development
'direct effects hypothesis' (social support) 20

'effort syndrome' 69–70
Emergence 128
emotional support 21
empowerment 62
environment and mental health 38–40
Erikson's stages of development 34–6

European Federation
    of Therapeutic
    Communities (EFTC)
    111
evaluating sessions 100–1
evidence base for mutual
    support 81–90

facilitator roles 18, 97
Families Anonymous 128
Finchden Manor (Kent)
    68
finding a mutual support
    group 94
    contact details 127–9
Foucalt, Michel 107
Foulkes, Sigmund 69, 86
Francis Dixon Lodge
    (Leicester) 90, 115

Garden Villa (Scotland)
    115
ground rules for groups
    98
group 'rules' 98
group structures (mutual
    support) 99–100
group therapy 55–6
    curative factors 56–8
    forms and types 58–64
    key benefits 55–8
    see also mutual support/
        groups; therapeutic
        communities

Haven Project (Colchester)
    115
health professionals
    see mental health
    professionals
Hearing Voices Network
    129
help-seeking behaviours
    45–7
helper-therapy principle
    22
helplessness 48

Henderson Hospital
    (Surrey) 70, 77,
    89–90
history of mental health
    service provisions
    48–52
    and therapeutic
        communities 65–7
HMP Units see prison
    units

identity, and social
    relationships 30–1
information sources
    109–30
    mutual support groups
        127–9
    professional
        organisations
        109–17
    therapeutic
        communities (for
        addictions) 120–1
    therapeutic communities
        (for adult offenders)
        117–20
    therapeutic communities
        (for adult offenders
        with addiction
        problems) 121
    therapeutic
        communities (for
        children and young
        people) 122–6
    therapeutic communities
        (for people with
        learning difficulties)
        126–7
informational support 21
Institute of Group
    Analysis (IGA) 111
instrumental support 21
internal working
    model (IWM) of
    relationships 28, 30

Jones, Maxwell 69–70, 86

Lane, Homer 67–8
learning difficulties,
    therapeutic
    communities 126–7
legislation on mental
    health 50
    recent changes 53
Lothlorien (Scotland) 115
Lyward, George 68

McDonald Bell, George
    69
Macmillan, Duncan 69
Main, Tom 68–70, 86
Mandala Therapeutic
    Community
    (Nottingham) 116
Maudsley Hospital,
    Cawley Centre 113
Max Glatt Centre
    (Wormwood Scrubs)
    71–2
medical health
    practitioners 53
medical model (mental
    health services) 51–2,
    53–4
meetings
    planning considerations
        95–6
    venues 96
Mental Health Act–2007
    53, 105
mental health difficulties
    33–41
    contexts and trigger
        factors 11
    social relationships
        and attachments
        31–2
    socio-political
        37–41
    prevalence 38
    and psychosocial stages
        34–7

mental health
    professionals 18
    incorporating ideas into
        clinical practice
        102
    involvement in group
        work 92–4
    ways to provide support
        101
mental health services
    background and history
        48–52
    community-based care
        policies 40–1
    current provisions and
        approaches 52–4
    future implications for
        mutual support
        103–8
Mill Hill (London) 69–70
Mills, Hannah 49
'moral treatment' 49–50,
    66–7, 106
    decline 51
Mutual Aid: A Factor of
    Evolution (Kropotkin)
    24
mutual support/groups
    background and history
        60–1
    benefits of group
        therapy 55–8
    concept described
        17–23
    current perspectives 23
    definitions 18–19
    evidence base and
        research studies
        81–5
    future considerations
        103–8
    importance of
        professional
        involvement 92–4
    improving access 91–4
    key principles 61–3

lists of groups and
    contact details
    127–9
locating groups 94
pros and cons 93–4
reviewing group
    sessions 100–1
session planning 95–6
socio-political contexts
    37–41
standards and quality
    issues 74–7
structuring the group
    99–100
within therapeutic
    communities 87–90
see also social support;
    therapeutic
    communities

National Association for
    People Abused in
    Childhood (NAPAC)
    129
NIMHE 77
normalisation processes
    62
Northfield Military
    Hospital
    (Birmingham) 68–70

obsessive compulsive
    disorder support
    groups 129

Peper Harow 68
personal identity 30–1
personality, stages of
    development 34–7
Personality Disorder: No
    Longer a Diagnosis of
    Exclusion (NIMHE) 77
PET see planned
    environment therapy
    (PET)
Philadelphia Association
    (London) 116
Pinel, Phillipe 49–50

Planned Environment
    therapy (PET) 67–8,
    111–12
planning sessions 95–6
power differentials in
    mental health 47–8,
    53
prevalence of mental
    health difficulties 38
prevention equation
    (Albee) 63
prison units 71–2
    adult therapeutic
        communities
        117–20
    therapeutic communities
        for adult with
        addictions 121
    professional involvement
        92–4
    ways to provide support
        101
professional organisations
    109–12
psychiatric profession,
    early developments
    51–2
psycho-educational groups
    58, 59–60
psychosocial stages of
    development 34–7
psychotherapy groups
    58, 59
publicity and advertising
    96–7

Quaker movement 49
quality issues 74–7

randomised controlled
    trials (RCTs) 83–4
Recovery Inc. 83
Red Hill School 68
Red House Psychotherapy
    Service (Manchester)
    116
refreshment provisions
    (support meetings) 98

rehabilitation, early concepts 66–7
research studies
  on mutual support 82–5
  on therapeutic communities 85–90
Responsible Clinician (RC) 53
Rethink 129
The Retreat *see* The York Retreat
reviewing group sessions 100–1
'revolving door' phenomenon 40–1
Richmond Fellowship 116
role models 62, 99
Rose, Melvyn 68

schizophrenia, environmental effects 38–9
seeking help *see* help-seeking behaviours
The Self–Help Group Sourcebook (White and Madara) 61–3
Self-help groups, cf. mutual support groups 18
service provisions *see* mental health services
setting up a mutual support group 95–7
  facilitator roles 97
shared experiences 21–2
Shaw, Otto 68
social comparison theory 22
social factors and mental health 11–12, 37–41
  environmental influences 38–40
social nature of humans 24–5
social networks 39

social support
  background and literature 19–20
  benefits 20
  cf. mutual support 19
  definitions 19–20
socio-political factors and mental health 37–41
stages of development *see* psychosocial stages of development
standards of care 74–7
stigma and mental health 10
  impact on help-seeking behaviours 46
'Strange Situation' (Ainsworth *et al.*) 26
'stress-buffering hypothesis' (social support) 20
Summerhill School 68
support groups
  cf. mutual support groups 18–19
  see also mutual support/ groups; therapeutic communities
supportive interactions 20–2
  forms and types 21
  principles and theories 22
  shared experiences 21–2

therapeutic communities 65–74
  background and history 65–7
  common attributes 73–4
  concepts and theoretical basis 10–11, 65–6, 70–2
  current models and approaches 73–4
  described 10–11

  for adult offenders 117–20
  for adults (general) 112–17
  for children and young people 122–6
  for people with addictions 120–1
  for people with learning difficulties 126–7
  research and evidence base 85–90
  role of mutual support 87–90
  role within current healthcare system 76–7
  standards of care 74–7
Therapeutic Communities of America (TCA) 112
Threshold Services 116–17
transactional model of stress (Lazarus) 20
trust building 97–8
Tuke, Samuel 49–50

UK Narcotics Anonymous 129
United States, therapeutic communities 112

venues for meetings 96

Winterbourne House (Berks) 117
World Federation of Therapeutic Communities (WFTC) 112
Wormwood Scrubs 71–2

The York Retreat 49–50, 51, 52, 66, 112
young adults and children, therapeutic communities 122–6

Author Index

Ainsworth, M.D.S. 26
Albee, George 63
Albus, K.E. 32

Barker, C. 19, 45
Barrera, M. 20
Barrett, L. 24
Bartholomew, K. 31
Bebbington, P.E. 46
Bender, E. 18–19
Bennett, T.L. 20
Berke, J.H. 87
Biggs, V. 87–8
Bion, W.R. 69, 86
Bloom, J.R. 20
Borkman, T.J. 60
Bowlby, J. 25–32
Broekaert, E. 72
Brown, L.D. 84

Campling, P. 90
Carlson, E.A. 30
Cassel, J. 19
Chien, W.T. 84
Clark, D.H. 69–70
Coates, D. 22
Cobb, S. 19
Cohen, S. 19–20
Collins, M. 65–6
Collis, M. 86–7
Cook, J.A. 84
Corrigan, P.W. 38
Cowen, E.L. 46
Cross, D.G. 46
Cutrona, C.E. 19, 21

Davies, S. 90
Davison, K.P. 60–1
De Leon, G. 88
Dermatis, H. 88
Dickerson, S.S. 60–1
Dietrich, D. 31
Dolan, B.M. 89–90
Dooley, D. 20
Dozier, M. 32
Drahorad, C. 87
Dunbar, R. 24
Dunkel-Schetter, C. 20, 22

Edmunson, E.D. 83
Egeland, B. 30
Erikson, E. 34–6

Festinger, L. 22
Foulkes, S.R. 69, 86

Galanter, M. 83
Glatt, M.M. 71–2
Goldberg, D. 46
Goldstrom, I.D. 82–3
Goodman, G. 23
Gottlieb, B.H. 21
Grant, C. 84

Haaga, D.A.F. 46
Haigh, R. 72, 73–6, 90
Hancher-Kvam, S. 36
Helgeson, V.S. 19, 21–2
Heller, T. 84
Hogan, B. 20, 21
Horowitz, L.M. 31–2

House, J. 19
Humphreys, K. 18, 19, 83
Huxley, P. 46

Jablensky, A. 39
Jacobs, M.K. 23
Jones, M. 69–70, 86

Kahn, J.A. 46
Katz, A. 18–19
Kelly, J.F. 85
Kennard, D. 50–1, 65, 67–8
Kessler, R.C. 23
Kooyman, M. 72
Kropotkin, P. 24
Kurtz, L.F. 83
Kyrouz, E. 83

Labrecque, M.S. 84
Laing, R.D. 72
Landis, S.A. 19
Lazarus, R.S. 20
Lees, J. 72, 86
Lieberman, M.A. 21
Linden, W. 20
Lloyd, C. 31
Loat, M. 88–9
Loomis, C. 83
Lycett, J. 24
Lyons, J.S. 36

Madara, E.J. 61–3
Main, M. 26
Main, T.F. 68–70, 86
Mäkikyro, T. 31

Manning, N. 86
Masoliver, C. 87
Maton, K.I. 22, 62
Mickelson, K.D. 22, 23
Mind 34
Morris, M. 71

Najarian, B. 20
Neill, A.S. 68
NIMHE 77
Norman, I. 84

Osborn, M. 88
Ottenberg, D. 72

Penn, D.L. 38
Pennebaker, H.W. 60–1
Perotta, P. 36
Peters-Golden, H. 22
Pickett-Schenk, S.A. 84
Pierce, G.R. 19–20
Pinel, Phillipe 49–50
Pines, M. 58
Pistrang, N. 19, 45, 84

Rappaport, J. 18, 86
Rawlings, B. 86
Rees, T.P. 69
Richardson, L. 88
Riessman, F. 22, 61–2
Roberts, L.J. 22, 62, 83
Robertson, J. 25–6
Rossiter, C.M. 84
Ryan, K. 90
Ryan, T. 87

Sarason, B.R. 19–20
Sarason, I.G. 19–20
Sartorius, N. 39
Schlapobersky, J. 58
Shapiro, R. 39
Sheehan, P.W. 46
Silverman, P. 63
Skilton, L. 39
Smith, J.A. 88
Solomon, J. 26
Spiegel, D. 85

Sroufe, L.A. 30
Stovall, K.C. 32

Taylor, S.E. 19
Thompson, D.R. 84
Toro, P.A. 18
Toseland, R.W. 84
Trivedi, P. 53

Umberson, D. 19

White, B.J. 61–3
Whiteley, J.S. 65–6, 86–7
Willig, C. 88
Wills, W.D. 67–8
Wills, T.A. 20
Winston, T. 22
World Health
    Organization (WHO)
    38–9, 46
Wortman, C.B. 20

Yalom, I.D. 56–8

Zhao, S. 23

CPI Antony Rowe
Eastbourne, UK
December 06, 2019